Concepts in Fetal
Movement Research

Concepts in Fetal Movement Research

Joyce W. Sparling
Editor

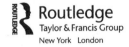

Routledge
Taylor & Francis Group
New York   London

Concepts in Fetal Movement Research has also been published as *Physical & Occupational Therapy in Pediatrics*, Volume 12, Numbers 2/3 1993.

First published by:

The Haworth Press, Inc., 10 Alice Street, Binghamton, NY 13904-1580, USA

This edition published 2011 by Routledge:

Routledge
Taylor & Francis Group
711 Third Avenue
New York, NY 10017

Routledge
Taylor & Francis Group
2 Park Square, Milton Park
Abingdon, Oxon OX14 4RN

Library of Congress Cataloging-in-Publication Data

Concepts in fetal movement research / Joyce W. Sparling, editor.
     p. cm.
    "Has also been published as Physical & occupational therapy in pediatrics, volume 12, numbers 2/3 1993"–T.p. verso.
    Includes bibliographical references and index.
    ISBN 1-56024-449-6 (h : alk. paper)
    1. Fetus–Movements. 2. Fetus–Imaging. I. Sparling, Joyce W.
    [DNLM: 1. Fetal Movement. 2. Fetus. W1 PH683P v. 12 nos. 2/3 1993 / WQ 210 C7444 1992]
RG621.C66 1992
612.6'47–dc20
DNLM/DLC
for Library of Congress
                                    92-48442
                                       CIP

Concepts in Fetal Movement Research

CONTENTS

ABOUT THE EDITOR

Joyce Whitaker Sparling, PhD, PT, OT, received her AB degree in Psychology and Comparative Sciences from Wellesley College and her certificate in Physical Therapy from Duke University. Her interest in pediatric physical therapy was first stimulated by Nancy deWolf at the Meeting Street School in Providence, Rhode Island, and continued at Children's Hospital in Boston with Claire McCarthy and Elizabeth Zausmer, and later through consultation with Jan Wilson at United Cerebral Palsy and Lenox Baker Children's Hospital in Durham, NC. After twenty-two years as a clinician, she furthered her interest in life-span development, functional activities, and theory-based practice by obtaining a Master of Science degree in Occupational Therapy at the University of North Carolina with Joan Rogers. Her doctoral work on adaptation to prenatal diagnosis of impairment was conducted in Special Education at Frank Porter Graham Research Center with Dale Farran and Rune Simeonsson and was accomplished in collaboration with obstetricians John Seeds and Vern Katz. Further work with low-risk and high-risk fetuses was conducted with Irma Wilhelm, her colleague in Physical Therapy. Fetal movement and the adaptation of families to special needs children have become the focus of her research in the Division of Physical Therapy at the University of North Carolina at Chapel Hill.

Preface

The study of fetal movement is an exploration of human development to reveal some of its mysteries that have persisted throughout the first half of the twentieth century. This investigation is a multidimensional experience causing investigators to confront their ethical and cultural beliefs, as well as to question hypotheses about sensorimotor development, and to hone their observational skills. In addition, the study of fetal movement includes an evaluation of the environment of the fetus, and an attempt to understand subtle variations in that environment that may have profound effects on development. Fetal behavior reveals the confluence of endogenous and environmental factors.

Describing fetal movement characteristics requires a constant blending of observation and technology. In our attempts to observe aspects of fetal movement that are unique, we have been thrilled by the window that ultrasound technology has opened onto the fetus. The varying aspects of this technology have been effectively described in the paper by Dr. Vern Katz, who has been a supporter of fetal movement study since its inception at the University of North Carolina (UNC). Safety related to obstetric ultrasound imaging has been consistently questioned, as Tucker, Thomas, Gentry and Sparling describe. Although no apparent danger exists in the use of this technology, researchers in the United States are being diligent in regulating its use. At the same time that we are enraptured by views of the fetus, we are dismayed by the two-dimensional nature of ultrasound and the half-tones of the gray scale. The diffuse quality of some body part outlines, the variability of the depth of focus, and the frequent optical distortion are obstacles to gaining high interrater reliability in assessing real-time movement. Even slight movement of the transducer, fetus or mother can impede the reliable scoring of real-time observations.

Researchers have experienced difficulty in kinematic measurement of fetal movement, yet we have the initial work of Audrey Macdonald in Canada and Cheryl Riegger-Krugh at UNC to prove that it can be done. Professor Macdonald's research on scapular movements at 20 weeks attests to the precision that is possible. So too does the research of Dr. Riegger-Krugh who is determining fetal segmental masses and measuring angular velocities of fetal leg movements in order to assess the force quality of those movements. The study of these researchers coupled with that of Sparling, Green, MacLeod, Wilhelm and Katz provides information relative to the structure versus function dialogue.

In Sparling, Green, MacLeod, Wilhelm and Katz's introductory article, the framework for fetal movement research has been outlined. The need for reliable assessment couched in a systems perspective is emphasized. Previous fetal movement research has facilitated discussion between researchers espousing the quantitative and qualitative approaches. The approach taken by the UNC group in developing assessment instruments (Sparling, Wilhelm and Green, Sparling) attests that both perspectives are necessary and offer different types of information in the measurement of fetal movement. The obvious factor limiting the quantitative approach is the visual clarity of the subject. Although obstetricians and radiologists can diagnose small neural tube and other specific defects, the analysis of movement of the fetus has been less straightforward, leading to the use of global descriptors to categorize human observations.

From the initiation of the UNC group's research on fetal movement, the continuity-discontinuity in movements and behavioral state over the birth transition has been an area of interest. Irma Wilhelm's review of literature on fetal state sets the stage for Long, McCusker, Ruble and Sparling's study of activity and inactivity in the young fetus. Ann Marie MacLeod has long been intrigued with the relationship between fetal and neonatal movement and has used Als' Synactive Theory to guide her study in this area.

The study of fetal movement as with any other intellectual effort is a collaborative labor. Interaction with Dr. Mecca Cranley, Dean of the School of Nursing at SUNY Buffalo, has been an ambition of mine since embarking on fetal research. Her perspectives on the attachment of mothers *and* fathers to their fetuses provides the social complement to the biologic perspective. In studying the dimensions of parental attachment to the fetus, she has identified a major psychological and social task of pregnancy. Dr. Ted Lyons has used his creative talents and imaging knowledge to gaze into the future and suggest what it holds for us in radiology and fetal movement research.

Directions pursued in our work were derived from myriad discussions throughout the last four years. Numerous people along the way have shown enthusiasm for applying the physical therapist's knowledge base to this relatively untapped period of development. The authors of the enclosed papers want to thank all who shared in the development of their thought related to fetal study. A particular thanks is extended to Suzanne Davlin and Irma Wilhelm for their editorial assistance, to Ann Lauder for assistance with graphic design, and to Jackie O'Neal for her secretarial assistance and patience.

Our excursion into fetal movement research began with Dr. John Seeds, Dr. Rune Simeonsson and Dr. Dale Farran and has continued with Vern Katz, Irma Wilhelm, Sandra Green, and Ann Marie MacLeod. Strong support throughout the project has come from Jim Papai, Lib Brannon and the Maternal and Child Health Bureau of the Department of Health and Human Services, USPHS. The postgraduate training grant which UNC has received since 1966 created opportunities for sharing of perspectives and information with a diversity of persons. The professional insight and courtesy that these leaders have shown in fostering our development is deeply appreciated. Hopefully, this monograph will stimulate physical therapists and investigators in related fields to extend their leadership skills in the study of fetal movement.

Throughout our study, Ruth Mitchell has been a sounding board for discussion of the enormous ethical issues involved in this research. She has provided guidance and a principled perspective on investigation in this sensitive area. Special educators at Frank Porter Graham Child Development Center have supplied financial and intellectual support.

Administrative support from David Yoder and Darlene Sekerak has been forthcoming since the inception of this study. They continuously encouraged the pursuit of this area of investigation, supplying funding and space. Our laboratory has been essential for housing equipment, providing sanctuary, and offering a quiet environment in which to score hundreds of hours of videotape.

This monograph and the research efforts it describes would not exist without the women who willingly volunteered to have imaging at various times throughout their pregnancy. We thank you and dedicate this book to you.

Joyce Sparling
Editor
July 10, 1992

Concepts
in Fetal Movement Research

Joyce W. Sparling
Sandra Green
Ann Marie MacLeod
Irma J. Wilhelm
Vern L. Katz

SUMMARY. Through the use of ultrasound imaging, human fetal movement can be directly observed and assessed. This capability coupled with the expansion of neuroscientific knowledge and related theories has encouraged physical therapists, obstetricians, neurologists and radiologists to work together to explore the role of fetal movement in development. Directions for fetal movement study are suggested, based on this information, and guidelines for research consistent with the dynamical systems theory are presented.

Permeating Darwin's writings is his belief that observation and its detailed recording are critical to the advance of science. If observation is to be of value, however, it should be accompanied by speculation and result in some questions or hypotheses.[1] Through observation, concepts and ideas are formulated to generate hypotheses and through systematic data collection these hypotheses are ultimately confirmed or rejected. Observation is a common experience, yet as a research methodology it is not a simple process. Observation is not an approach located on one end of the research continuum of control or precision,[2,p39] but a complex systematic research methodology to assess and generate new ideas about reality.

This review was partially funded by a Maternal and Child Health Postgraduate Training Grant from the Department of Health and Human Services, USPHS.

1

Observational skills are required in the use of ultrasound technology for fetal imaging. With systematic observation of real-time fetal movement, hypotheses about early human movement can be developed. Confirmation of these hypotheses may need to await the further advancement of technology, but at the very least researchers in this area can gather data and speculate about the significance of early movement for motor development. Darwin's thesis, therefore, encouraging observation and speculation, is fundamental to fetal movement research. The purpose of this paper is to speculate on the meaning of activity and inactivity of young fetuses in their natural environment, to share neuroscientific research and hypotheses related to early neural development, and to lay the groundwork for clinical research on fetal movement. Studies of fetal movement in this monograph are placed in an historical perspective by reviewing early attempts to analyze movement. A further purpose is to establish an understanding of the implications of fetal movement study for the disciplines of physical and occupational therapy.

BACKGROUND OF FETAL MOVEMENT RESEARCH

Fetal movement has been noted since ancient times, but only recently have technology and movement theory been sufficiently developed to permit the direct observation of spontaneous fetal movement and speculate about its significance. Prior to the 1960's, the prominent theories directing studies of human and animal movement were reflexology and the hierarchical theory. Presently, the motor control theory prevails and describes coordinated movement as emerging from an interaction of the nervous system with other systems.[3] Just as theories of motor development have progressed, so too has technology advanced. In the mid 1970's, real-time ultrasound (US) was introduced into obstetric practice[4] and permitted observation of spontaneous fetal movement. The timely confluence of technology and theory development provided the permissive conditions for a number of European studies of spontaneous human movement. Specific details of these studies will be discussed. A more extensive review has been published by Cintas[5] and others.[6]

Theoretical Perspectives

Ironically, in the earliest clinical investigation,[7] Preyer described fetal movement as spontaneous in nature. Through observations of chick embryos, Preyer proposed a theory of motor primacy in which embryonic movement was assumed to be active rather than reactive. When discussing the genesis of movement, Preyer suggested that early motility was autogenous, in that the movement was generated in the interneurons and motor neurons of the spinal cord, and, therefore, that sensory information was not a prerequisite for early movement.

In the first part of this century, investigators[8,9] proposed reflexology as a theoretical perspective to guide future research. In later investigations espousing this perspective, recently aborted fetuses were stimulated and their reflex responses were recorded.[10-12] Researchers utilizing these methods assumed that motor patterns developed through the integration of local reflexes into coordinated patterns of movement.

Through the research of Hamburger in the 50s,[13] the significance of Preyer's early thinking was confirmed. Observing the chick embryo, Hamburger noted spontaneous leg movement on day six, while motor response to a stimulus did not occur until 7.5 days. The early appearance of spontaneous movement in the absence of afferent input suggested the presence of innate motor programs: centrally generated, intrinsic properties of the central nervous system. Evidence for the occurrence of innate motor patterns in the absence of afferent or supraspinal input has been provided by a number of investigators. Weiss[14] deafferented the lumbar region of frog tadpoles before the legs were functional. When the legs of the frog began to move, coordinated movement was not impaired. Weiss concluded that afferent information was not necessary for normal locomotion patterns. In further animal studies, investigators transected the spinal cord of various animals to eliminate supraspinal input. Hindlimb movements persisted after transection of the spinal cord in fetal kittens.[15] Transected and deafferented chick embryos exhibited hindlimb EMG patterns.[16] Muscle activation patterns were consistent with mature motor function with alternation of antagonistic muscles and co-activation of synergistic muscles. Further evidence for movement occurring in the absence of afferent input included research determining that the motor neuron connections to muscles are developed first, followed by interneurons to motor neurons, and last, by afferent connections to motor neurons.[12,17,18]

While movement can occur in the absence of afferent stimulation, afferent input does provide some central nervous system drive to initiate movement.[19] Afferent information also modulates some of the neural circuitry[20] to produce different output patterns. Walking and hatching movement patterns in chicks, for example, became more similar to one another after deafferentation.[19] Since the walking pattern became more like hatching, hatching was postulated as the more basic pattern. Although some disagreement remains among researchers about the existence and neural structure of these innate motor programs, many believe they are soft-wired and, therefore, they may be modified as well as modify other patterns.

Evidence from animal research initiated a change in the focus of research from examining elicited movement to describing spontaneous movement. The advent of ultrasound supported this change by providing the technology required for the naturalistic study of spontaneous fetal movement.

The Use of Ultrasound in Obstetric Research

The development of ultrasound (US) as a commercially available diagnostic tool revolutionized obstetric care and provided a research instrument permitting observation of real-time movement. According to Oakley,[21] US was initially developed during World War I to locate submarines. In the mid-1950's, industrial ultrasound equipment that was used for detecting flaws in metal was adopted to diagnose abdominal tumors. In 1973, US was first used to observe fetal movement.[4] Reinold's initial studies characterizing spontaneous movement described broad categories of movement.[22] In 1978, Birnholz, Stephens and Faria[10] described spontaneous movement via real time imaging, but used Hooker and Humphrey's reflex orientation for descriptors. The twitch, "a single gross episode of trunk flexion and head extension without separate or associated limb movement,"[10,p537] was the first movement noted around 7.5 weeks, while the last movement to appear was the "periodic repetitive movements of the diaphragm with simultaneous chest wall excursions"[10,p538] that were first noted at 24-28 weeks. These movements were interpreted within the framework of the earlier studies of elicited movement, but suggested the potential importance of US in the clinical management of pregnancy.[10]

The most extensive early investigation in terms of number of subjects was conducted by Ianniruberto and Tajani[23] who studied two thousand pregnant women from 8 to 41 weeks of gestation. Eighty-two of the 2000 subjects were systematically assessed weekly using imagings of 1 to 30 minutes duration. Motor patterns that were repeated consistently were categorized, but no durations or frequencies of the movement patterns were recorded. These investigators concluded that the repertoire of motor patterns was almost complete by 20 weeks gestation, and that pattern itemization and categorization was by itself an inadequate description because fetal motor patterns were so variable. As pioneers in this area of research, Ianniruberto and Tajani did much to stimulate interest in the study of human fetal movement.

Milani Comparetti[24] used a different method of pattern analysis to reanalyze data collected by Ianniruberto and Tajani. Milani Comparetti described the fetal movements as primary motor patterns (PMPs), and hypothesized that PMPs were genetically determined, intrinsic properties of the central nervous system that were partially independent of afferent information; in other words they were akin to innate motor programs. According to this perspective, PMPs have two categories: patterns that do or do not seem to have functional meaning. Primary motor patterns that seem to have functional meaning are called primary automatisms, while patterns that do not seem to have functional meaning are not further qualified. From all the patterns identified, Milani selected only primary automatisms for fetal observation.

Primary automatisms were hypothesized to have the following functions: (1) positioning for birth through fetal locomotion, (2) collaborating in labor through expression of the supporting reaction, (3) developing competencies for survival, such as rooting and sucking, and (4) developing competencies for emerging behaviors such as head postural control. Milani Comparetti did not provide a description of the PMPs, making comparisons between PMPs and patterns described by other investigators difficult. According to Milani Comparetti, a full repertoire of primary automatisms was present by 20 weeks gestation.

Based on this research, deVries, Visser and Prechtl[25] studied movement patterns during the early period of gestation, from 7 to 19 weeks postmenstrual age. Eleven healthy nulliparous women received 60 minutes of US weekly from 7 to 15 weeks and at 16 or 17 and 18 or 19 weeks gestational age. From this data, 16 fetal movement patterns closely resembling those observed in preterm and full term infants were distinguished. Fourteen of these 16 movement patterns were contained within Ianniruberto and Tajani's classification. Some of these qualifiers are compared in the paper by Green and Sparling in this issue.

deVries et al. observed that all movement patterns were present by 15 weeks of gestation.[25] The earlier time for initial pattern expression was determined because of the longer 60-minute observation periods, and the use of videotaped US recordings rather than live ultrasound imaging, as described by Ianniruberto and Tajani. In two subsequent papers, deVries, Visser and Prechtl analyzed recordings of the same 11 subjects for quantitative aspects of fetal behavior[26] and for individual differences and consistencies.[27] With a few exceptions, three age trends were found in the original 16 patterns:[26] (1) a gradual increase in incidence of breathing movements, head rotation, jaw opening, sucking and swallowing, a result suggesting a potential increase in organization of the fetus over time; (2) an increase followed by a decrease in the incidence of startles at 9 weeks, a decrease of hiccups at 13 weeks, and a decrease of retroflexion of the head at 12 weeks; and, (3) an increase in incidence of "general movements" until a plateau was reached at 10 weeks. General movements (GMs) were described as "gross movements involving the whole body . . . lasting from a few seconds to a minute . . . with a variable sequence of arm, leg, neck and trunk movements. They wax and wane in intensity, force and speed, and their onset and end are gradual . . . creating the impression of complexity and variability."[28,pp152-153]

Recently, Hadders-Algra and Prechtl[29] have described a transition period in these GMs that occurs postnatally around two months. At this time, the GMs are transformed from "writhing" movements noted in the fetus to "fidgety" movements in the neo-nate. The transformation is more consistent with postmenstrual age than with postnatal age suggesting an endogenous process. Because healthy preterm infants who received environmental stimulation displayed the fidgety movements earlier than full term infants, the authors also suggest the importance of exogenous influences on the developmental process.

Most of the fetal studies have been hampered by the lack of established reliability. Problems in achieving interrater reliability on randomly selected US imagings are discussed in the paper by Sparling and Wilhelm in this issue. Given the two-dimensional nature of US, the difficulty in achieving reliability is not surprising. Considering this significant limitation, the question that might appropriately be asked, is whether any purpose can be served by the study of human fetal movement at this time.

RATIONALE FOR FETAL MOVEMENT RESEARCH

Previous theories have described the process of motor development as apparently originating at birth. Gesell and Ilg's[30] observations depicting motor development from 0-60 postnatal weeks is a particularly vivid reminder of this phase of our research heritage. From the previous discussion, however, it is clear that human movement originates in the very young fetus. The purpose of this early movement for the fetus has been explained by three perspectives:[31] the epiphenomenal, functional, and preparatory views.

The Epiphenomenal View

Proponents of this view assume that fetal behaviors do not have adaptive significance. Fetal movement is interpreted as accidental to structural development, a result of neural maturation that lacks biological significance during the prenatal period. Support for this view was at its height during the periods when reflexology was the pervading theory of nervous system development. In perioral stimulation of exteriorized fetuses, Humphrey[9] described the primiti e reflexive status of the fetus by exhibiting rooting and other primitive reflexes.

The Functional View

Contradicting the epiphenomenal view, proponents of the functional view assume that fetal movement plays a significant role in the survival and development of the fetus. Specific movement patterns may serve to position the fetus for birth or assist with fetal collaboration in labor, as emphasized by Milani Comparetti.[24] Spontaneous movement may also ensure normal muscle and bone growth, a perspective elaborated upon by Riegger-Krugh in this issue. Prolonged immobilization of chick embryos[32] and of humans,[33] for example, has resulted in joint defects and growth retardation.

The Preparatory View

Persons favoring the preparatory hypothesis assume that the practice of movement patterns is crucial for the development of motor coordination and organization of postnatal behavior,[34] a primary principle of motor control theory. Through repetition of movement, fetuses may exhibit coordinated movement that suggests behavioral organization, as the functional view also demonstrates. Proponents of this view believe that fetal movement is necessary for subsequent behavioral and morphological development. Motor patterns emerge early in prenatal development and are repeated until the patterns fulfill a meaningful task as part of a complex adaptive function. Jeka and Kelso suggest, however, that "until we understand these systems better, we should probably resist ascribing a priori the process of pattern selection to an agency residing inside the system."[35,pp36-37]

Elements of the functional and preparatory views have been incorporated in contemporary fetal research. Our perspective embraces these views but extends them to specifically include general systems and related theories of motor control. Unlike present studies guided by systems thinking, however, the inaccessibility of the fetus for direct study limits the type of data that can be collected.

APPLICATION OF DYNAMIC SYSTEMS THEORY

Several dynamic systems concepts give direction to contemporary fetal movement research. Stability is both an environmental and a temporal factor used to describe a system in equilibrium. The process of change from stability to instability, and back to stability, is an essential characteristic of the developing organism. Environments that provide permissive conditions, restraints or challenges to the organism, foster change. The conditions of the task and the environment in which the task occurs interact to affect motor behavior. Specific functional tasks are repeated that support survival and development.

Stability and Change

The loss of stability is the "chief mechanism that effects a change pattern."[35,p14] This principle has been well expressed by Prigogene and Stengers,[36,p178] descriptions of "order through fluctuation" and has been applied to many fields including education,[37] and to families in transition,[38] as well as to the development of coordinated movement.[35] Instability, fluctuation, and change are characteristic processes of complex human systems.

The transition from the intrauterine to the extrauterine environment, with the concurrent experience of gravity and air exchange, is a major challenge for the human organism. When the conditions are supportive, the process of birth and adaptation to a new environment are accomplished and the organism achieves a more complex level of performance. Imagine the challenges in infancy: to stand with added weight and attempt to reciprocate; to become symmetrical and bring hands to midline for manipulation; and to interact with strangers as well as parents. These challenges thrust the infant temporarily into disequilibrium until new and stable states can be achieved.

Challenges exist for the fetus as well. The uterine environment is constantly changing: amniotic fluid levels increase throughout the first two trimesters, then level off, and then rapidly decrease; the umbilical cord is ever present as a toy as well as a lifeline; and sometimes amniotic bands appear and offer additional restraints and challenges. Many of the conditions that foster fetal development appear to be related to environmental factors.

Environment

Permissive conditions, such as physical support, encourage the achievement of functional outcomes for the system.[39] Identification of existing permissive conditions in the fetus, such as amniotic fluid levels, can help us understand appropriate and inappropriate challenges to the system. Those challenges that are just right for the individual create temporary instability and foster the development and expression of further competencies.

While "boundary conditions"[35] for the fetus may be identified as preexisting conditions such as maternal diabetes, amniotic fluid density and composition, or uterine size and contractile characteristics, permissive and restrictive conditions also include drugs and nutritional factors that accompany drug use, and the emotional environment created by parents for their developing fetus. Attachment of parent to fetus, described by Cranley in this issue, is a major force by which the environment influences the developing organism. In addition, breathing movements are affected by the change in environmental conditions from the fetal to the neonatal period.[41]

Early Coordination

The task of research is to determine "how the motor system is organized to produce coordinated action."[41,p179] Research on coordinative structures or movement synergies suggests that the neuromuscular apparatus is present earlier than the behavior it supports, and the presence of the permissive conditions encourages the emergence of the synergistic movement pattern. Clark and colleagues[39] noted that when physical support was extended to the newly walking infants, the interlimb coordination in infant gait more closely resembled the adult pattern. Thelen, Skala and Kelso[41] determined that with 6-week old infants, synergies exist even though their timing is not skilled as in the adult. When one leg was weighted, the kicking of that leg was disturbed and movement was slower, while the kick pattern of the unweighted leg was increased. This perturbation demonstrated the presence of early synergies in the legs that were coupled.

Early coordination has been observed in the alternation of leg movements against the uterine wall.[23] Determination of early synergies and the conditions that foster them, could add to the understanding of the development of coordinated movement in preterm as well as full term infants.

DIRECTIONS FOR FETAL STUDY

Current areas of research on movement coordination and control are of particular interest to the study of fetal movement and include the continuum of behavioral competency,[24,29,40,42,43] the relationship of parents to their fetus and infant,[44,45] the development of neural circuitry,[46] the role of strengthening and practice,[47] and the physiological stability of the fetus and neonate.[43,48] Specific therapeutic goals outlined by Heriza,[46,pp122-123] and consistent with these areas of research on motor coordination, have stimulated our thinking related to the fetus. They are the following: promotion of function, identification of transitions, manipulation of control parameters such as behavioral state or strength, modification of the environment, practice, and emphasis on process rather than outcomes.

Building on some of these ideas, research questions have been formulated. The initial need identified was for assessment instruments to record the complexity of early fetal movement patterns: one assessment has been inductively formulated by Sparling and Wilhelm, while the other has been deductively developed by Green and Sparling. From its inception, our fetal study has emphasized a broad systems perspective with our researchers applying experience gained in neonatal intensive care, analysis of dance movement, musculoskeletal assessment, family dynamics and in obstetrical practice. These experiences have enriched the team interaction, permitted skilled multisystem observation, and encouraged speculation.

Assessment development has emphasized the young fetus during motor pattern development. Fetal movements can be observed and related to current knowledge of the developing nervous system. Perhaps some of the chaotic movements we have observed are not necessarily "disorganized" but may derive from an underlying simple system.[35] The instability of early fetal movement might simply reflect an underlying simplicity of the early neural mechanisms. On the other hand, the chaotic patterns may reflect underlying chaotic systems, or deviation amplifying systems,[38,p248] in which a small input may produce a wide distribution and timing of observed behaviors. Other neuronal factors participate in and complicate the difficult interpretation of fetal movements. Neurons and their synapses are known to experience selective disintegration during the developmental process.[49,50] The exact timing of this occurrence is unknown, but observations suggest that a critical period may occur between 14 and 16 postmenstrual weeks, as described in the paper in this issue by Sparling and Wilhelm. Further observation is needed to support this speculation.

During the development of the assessments, different research approaches have been suggested. One approach to fetal movement study is to recognize pregnancy as a naturally occurring experience and simply observe in a systematic way, with appropriate and reliable tools, the behavior of the fetus, the context in which the fetus moves, and the interaction of the family with the fetus. Observation of this sort should be longitudinal in nature and address the continuity of competency across the birth transition, or across the more important transition suggested around two months of infancy.[29,42] This approach has been used to some degree by Prechtl's group with neurologists and obstetricians working collaboratively across the birth transition.

Another approach to fetal movement research may be to identify consistently occurring movement patterns, whether they be called innate motor programs, PMP's, or soft-wired patterns, and determine their stability over time through an assessment of fetal activity and inactivity. Determination of the dimensions of transition periods between specific activities and states or their precursors could follow. Only then could appropriate intervention be explored. Initial detailed assessment would enable us to understand when to either perturb the fetus or effect practice of motor behaviors leading to improved behavioral organization of the fetus and infant. This approach is now technically possible using acoustic stimulation applied to the mother's abdomen for brief periods.

Results of one study using an external electronic artificial larynx with women in the last four weeks of a normal pregnancy indicated the importance of fetal state prior to application of the stimulus.[51] The authors concluded that previous interpretations of acoustic stimulation as a disorganizer of states may be incorrect and that in some cases the stimulus can act as an organizer of state depending upon the state in which the fetus was initially perturbed. The appearance of gross body movements after vibroacoustic stimulation has ranged from 10[51] to 60[52] minutes suggesting a need for further investigation of the effect of such a stimulus on the nervous system.

A more tempered use of technology was described in a study[53] in which over one thousand women were evaluated on their perception of their fetuses' movement following an application of external vibroacoustic stimulation. Ninety-two percent of the women felt fetal movement upon stimulation and had the anticipated reactive non-stress test (NST). Of the 88 fetuses in the last four weeks of gestation whose mothers did not feel movement, 10 had a nonreactive NST. Of these 10, four were growth-retarded fetuses, had low Apgar scores, and required Cesarean sections, three experienced neonatal death, one was stillborn, and one was a neonate with cerebral palsy. One had reduced fetal movements for which labor was induced, but had a normal vaginal delivery, and was healthy. This study suggests an opportunity for therapists to become involved in collaborative projects to determine the least invasive type of prenatal intervention for encouraging functional pattern repetition for some at-risk fetuses.

GUIDELINES FOR RESEARCH

According to the dynamical systems approach, the "challenge for the therapist is to identify functional goals in motor tasks and to adapt environmental constraints to reduce the degrees of freedom that must be controlled by the nervous system."[3,p17] We can apply this postnatal dictum to the prenatal period by identifying external factors or permissive conditions that allow the expression of functional motor patterns and challenge the fetus to vary the expression and timing of these patterns. Modifying the type or level of activity of the mother might alter physiological mechanisms affecting the fetus, as described by Katz[54] who studied pregnant women exercising in water. Modifying the density of the amniotic fluid, for example, might provide increased resistance to movements and facilitate strengthening of certain fetuses to better prepare them for the birthing process. On another level, providing appropriate information in a sensitive manner is a more realistic and immediate approach that could enhance maternal and paternal attachment to their fetus. This approach is discussed in detail by Cranley in this issue.

In observing the developing fetus, we are witnesses to the developmental tasks that need to be accomplished within a specific environment to achieve order out of instability, and to control the enormous degrees of freedom available to the fetus.[55] Many of the movement patterns appear to be brought under some control through the mechanism of fetal uterine constraints. The uterine wall offers a stable surface to the fetus for pushing off the uterine contour into leg extension, for thrusting into the wall with its head in preparation for cervical extension during birth, and for molding to the wall during periods of inactivity. The umbilical cord can be explored, grasped and pulled. These environmental opportunities foster fetuses to self-organize. Sparling and Wilhelm have described these characteristic fetal movements in their assessment in this issue. Interpreted within a dynamical systems perspective, legs are often in "brace" patterns that could be described as point attractor movements,[46,p109] while arms reach to grasp the cord or body part and exhibit a point attractor pattern. Other early leg movements appear to be collaborative in that one leg moves in the periodic or limit cycle trajectory, while the other leg moves in the point trajectory pattern, with one leg maintaining the trunk in some stability while the contralateral leg circumducts. The ability to uncouple and then repeat these leg movements might suggest the presence of enhanced behavioral organization, preparing fetuses for the birthing process and the extrauterine challenge of gravity.

In clinical practice, therapists attempt to identify variables that foster a resolution of transitional instability and achieve motor equilibrium. A further therapeutic challenge that is used by some therapists, is the identification of variables that help to create disequilibrium, thus encouraging self-organizing behavior. Basic to both approaches is the recognition of the importance of environmental manipulation.

In observing fetal movement, most research questions regarding the fetus will of necessity involve an ethical component. The researcher needs an awareness of the issues and a concern for the social relevancy of the research. The questions related to the high fetal and infant mortality rate in this country[56] are not separate issues, but need to be addressed in the conduct of all studies with pregnant women.

REFERENCES

1. Darwin CG. *On the Origin of Species by Means of Natural Selection.* New York: The Heritage Press; 1963.

2. Fassnacht G. *Theory and Practice of Observing Behaviour.* New York, NY: Academic Press;1982.

3. Horak FB. Assumptions underlying motor control for neurologic rehabilitation, In: Foundation for Physical Therapy. *Contemporary Management of Motor Control Problems. Proceedings of the II Step Conference.* Fredericksburg, VA: Bookcrafters, Inc.; 1991:11-27.

4. Reinold E. Clinical value of fetal spontaneous movements in early pregnancy. *J Perinatol Med.* 1973;1:65-69.

5. Cintas HM. Fetal movements: an overview. *Phys Occup Ther Pediatr.* 1987;7(3):1-15.

6. Tuck SM. Ultrasound monitoring of fetal behaviour. *Ultrasound Med Biol.* 1986;12(4):307-317.

7. Preyer W. *Spezielle Physiologie des Embryo.* Leipzig; Grieben:1985.

8. Swenson EA. The development of movement of albino rats before birth. Unpublished doctoral dissertation. Lawrence, KA: University of Kansas;1926. Dissertation.

9. Windle WF, Orr DW. The development of behavior in chick embryos: spinal cord structure correlated with early somatic motility. *J Comp Neurol.* 1934; 60:287-308.

10. Hooker D. *The Prenatal Origin of Behavior.* 18th Porter Lecture. Lawrence, KA: University of Kansas Press;1952.

11. Humphrey T. Function of the nervous system during prenatal life, In: Stave V, ed. *Perinatal Physiology.* New York, NY: Plenum:1978;651-683.

12. Birnholz JC, Stephens JC, Faria M. Fetal movement patterns: a possible means of defining neurological developmental milestones in utero. *Am J Roentgenol.* 1978;130:537-540.

13. Hamburger V. Some aspects of the embryology of behavior. *Quart Rev Biol.* 1963;38:342-365.

14. Weiss P. Does sensory control play a constructive role in the development of motor coordination? *Schweiz Med Wochenschr.* 1941;12:591-595.

15. Brown TG. On the activities of the central nervous system of the unborn fetus of the cat: with a discussion of the question whether progression is a "learnt" complex. *J Physiol.* (London). 1915;49:208-215.

16. Landmesser LT, O'Donovan MJ. Activation patterns of embryonic chick hindlimb muscles recorded in ovo and in an isolated spinal cord preparation. *J Physiol.* 1984;347:189-204.

17. Okado N. Onset of synapse formation in the human spinal cord. *J Comp Neurol.* 1981;201:211-219.

18. Saito K. Development of spinal reflexes in the rat fetus studied in vitro. *J Physiol.* (London). 1979;294:581-594.

19. Bekoff A, Sabichi AL. Sensory control of the initiation of hatching in chicks: effects of a local anesthetic injected into the neck. *Dev Psychobiol.* 1987;20(5):489-495.

20. Bekoff A, Nusbaum MP, Sabichi AL, Clifford M. Neural control of limb coordination. 1. comparison for hatching and walking output patterns in normal and deafferented chicks. *J Neurosci.* 1987;7(8):2320-2330.

21. Oakley A. The history of ultrasonography in obstetrics. *Birth.* 1986;13:8-13.

22. Reinold E. Ultrasonics in early pregnancy, diagnostic scanning and fetal motor activity. *Contrib Gynaecol Obstet.* 1976;1:103-127.

23. Ianniruberto A, Tajani E. Ultrasonographic study of fetal movements. *Semin Perinatol.* 1982;5(2):175-181.

24. Milani Comparetti A. The neurophysiologic and clinical implications of studies on fetal motor behavior. *Semin Perinatol.* 1981;5(2):183-189.

25. deVries JIP. Visser GHA, Prechtl HFR. The emergence of fetal behavior, I.Qualitative aspects. *Early Hum Dev.* 1982;7:301-322.

26. deVries JIP, Visser GHA, Prechtl HFR. The emergence of fetal behavior. II.Quantitative aspects. *Early Hum Dev.* 1985;12:99-120.

27. deVries JIP, Visser GHA, Prechtl HFR. The emergence of fetal behavior. III. Individual differences and consistencies. *Early Hum Dev.* 1988;16:85-103.

28. Prechtl HFR. Qualitative changes of spontaneous movements in fetus and preterm infant are a marker of neurological dysfunction. *Early Hum Dev.* 1990; 23:151-158.

29. Hadders-Algra M, Prechtl HFR. Developmental course of general movements in early infancy. I. descriptive analysis of change in form. *Early Hum Dev.* 1992;28:201-213.

30. Gesell A, Ilg FL. *Child Development: An Introduction to the Study of Human Growth.* New York, NY: Harper & Brothers;1943:224-237.

31. Oppenheim RW. Ontogenetic adaptations and retrogressive processes in the development of the nervous system and behavior: A neuroembryological perspective, In: Connolly KJ, Prechtl HFR, eds. *Maturation and Development: Biological and Psychological Perspectives.* Philadelphia, PA: Lippincott;1981:73-109.

32. Drachman DB, Sokoloff L. The role of movement in embryonic joint formation. *Dev Biol.* 1966;14:401-420.

33. Smith DW. *Recognizable Patterns of Human Deformation: Identification and Management of Mechanical Effects on Morphogenesis.* Philadelphia, PA: WB Saunders Company;1981.

34. Bekoff M, Byuers JA, Bekoff A. Prenatal motility and postnatal play: Functional continuity? *Dev Psychobiol.* 1980;13:225-228.

35. Jeka JJ, Kelso JAS. The dynamic pattern approach to coordinated behavior: a tutorial review. In: Wallace SA, ed. *Perspectives on the Coordination of Movement*. New York, NY: Elsevier Science Publishers;1989:3-45.

36. Prigogine I, Stengers I. *Order Out of Chaos: Man's New Dialogue with Nature*. New York, NY:Bantam Books;1984.

37. Sawada D, Caley MT. Dissipative structures. *Educ Res*. 1985; March:13-19.

38. Gottman JM. Chaos and regulated change in families: a metaphor for the study of transitions. In: Cowan PA, Hetherington M, eds. *Family Transitions*. Hillsdale, NJ: Lawrence Erlbaum Associates; 1991:247-272.

39. Clark JE, Whitall J, Phillips SJ. Human interlimb coordination: the first 6 months of independent walking. *Dev Psychobiol*. 1988;21(5):445-456.

40. Prechtl HFR. *Continuity and Change in Early Neural Development. Clinics in Developmental Medicine*. Philadelphia, PA: Lippincott;1984:1-14.

41. Thelen E, Skala KD, Kelso JAS. The dynamic nature of early coordination: evidence from bilateral leg movements in young infants. *Dev Psychol*. 1987; 23(2):179-186.

42. Robertson SS. Human cyclic motility: fetal-newborn continuities and newborn state differences. *Dev Psychobiol*. 1987;20(4): 425-442.

43. Als H. Toward a synactive theory of development: promise for the assessment and support of infant individuality. *Infant Mental Health J*. 1982;3:229-243.

44. Cranley M. Roots of attachment: the relationship of parents with their unborn. *Birth Defects*. 1981;17(6):59-83.

45. Sparling JW, Seeds JW, Farran DC. The relationship of obstetric ultrasound to parent and infant behavior. *Obstet Gynecol*. 1988;72:902-907.

46. Heriza C. Motor development: traditional and contemporary theories. In: Foundation for Physical Therapy. *Contemporary Management of Motor Control Problems. Proceedings of the II Step Conference*. Fredericksburg, VA: Bookcrafters, Inc.; 1990;99-126.

47. Shea AM. Motor attainments in Down Syndrome. In: Foundation for Physical Therapy. *Contemporary Management of Motor Control Problems. Proceedings of the II Step Conference*. Fredericksburg, VA: Bookcrafters, Inc.; 1990:225-236.

48. Hume RF, O'Donnell KJ, Stanger CL, Killam AP, Gingras JL. In utero cocaine exposure: observations of fetal behavioral state may predict neonatal outcome. *Am J Obstet Gynecol*. 1989;161:685-690.

49. Purves D, Lichtman JW. Elimination of synapses in the developing nervous system. *Science*. 1980;210:153-157.

50. Herschkowitz N. Brain development in the fetus, neonate and infant. *Biol Neonate*. 1988; 54:1-19.

51. Devoe LD, Murray C, Faircoloth D, Ramos E. Vibroacoustic stimulation and fetal behavioral state in normal term human pregnancy. *Am J Obstet Gynecol*. 1990;163:1156-1161.

52. Gagnon R, Hunse C, Carmichael L, Fellows F, Patrick J. Effects of vibratory acoustic stimulation on human fetal breathing and gross fetal body movements near term. *Am J Obstet Gynecol*. 1986;155:1227-1230.

53. Arulkumaran S, Anandakumar C, Wong YC, Ratnam SS. Evaluation of maternal perception of sound-evoked fetal movement as a test of antenatal fetal health. *Obstet Gynecol.* 1989;73:182-186.

54. Katz VL, McMurray R, Goodwin WE, Cefalo RC. Nonweightbearing exercise during pregnancy on land and during immersion: a comparative study. *Am J Perinatol.* 1990;7(3):281-284.

55. Thelen E, Ulrich BD. *Hidden Skills.* Monographs of the Society for Research in Child Development, Serial No.223. 1991: 56(1).

56. US Department of Health & Human Services. *Healthy Children 2000.* Washington, DC;DHHS No.HRSA-M-CH 91-2.

Relationship of Mechanical
and Movement Factors
to Prenatal Musculoskeletal Development

Cheryl Riegger-Krugh

SUMMARY. Physical and occupational therapists analyze mechanical forces and movement to understand human musculoskeletal dysfunction. Based on this analysis, therapists impose mechanical forces and movement on patients during intervention in order to normalize musculoskeletal tissues. The direct imposition of these forces on the fetus is limited, but the identification and analysis of them is an exciting area of exploration and research that may ultimately enhance intervention. The effects of these external and internal forces on the fetus are reviewed, and the areas of ongoing research at the University of North Carolina at Chapel Hill are discussed.

Knowledge of the effects of mechanical and movement factors on postnatal musculoskeletal development is greater than on prenatal development. Until recently, little emphasis has been placed on the study of these factors on fetal musculoskeletal development because of the inaccessibility of the fetus to direct and safe observation. Recent technical advances, however, have resulted in noninvasive study of fetal movement and related factors. The purposes of this article are to discuss the effects of mechanical and movement

Cheryl Riegger-Krugh, ScD, PT, is currently Assistant Professor, Division of Physical Therapy, University of North Carolina, Chapel Hill, NC 27599-7135.

Address for reprints: Division of Physical Therapy, CB#7135 Medical School Wing E, University of North Carolina at Chapel Hill, Chapel Hill, NC 27599-7135.

The author would like to express thanks and gratitude to Mary Clyde Singleton, PhD, PT, for helpful comments and suggestions.

factors on prenatal musculoskeletal development and share research methods and preliminary findings from several research projects involving the fetus.

The term "development" is used as a lifespan term to emphasize that a living being changes throughout life, and that there is value to life at different developmental stages.[1] Traditionally, development has meant embryonic, fetal and postnatal formation and growth to the age of maturity. The focus of this paper is on development during the embryonic (prenatal weeks 2-8) and fetal (prenatal weeks 9-birth) periods. Mechanical forces will be distinguished as forces imposed that are external to the fetus (external forces) and forces applied within the fetus (internal forces). Movement can include large scale, visible movement or small scale, subtle movement. More visible movement relates to joint motion, such as flexion, abduction, internal rotation, or translation of the fetus as a whole. More subtle movement includes joint accessory motions (glides and spins), tissue or structure deformation or strain, and altered position of structures resulting from varying rates of differentiation in adjacent structures.

MUSCULOSKELETAL SYSTEM– MECHANICAL FORCE AND MOVEMENT

The musculoskeletal system includes skeletal muscle, bones, ligaments, tendons, cartilage, especially articular cartilage, and junctions among some of these structures. Of the four tissue types– muscle, connective tissue, epithelium, and nerve tissue–muscle and connective tissue are the primary tissues composing the structures of the musculoskeletal system. During prenatal musculoskeletal development, the effects of mechanical and movement factors primarily are on muscle and connective tissues.

Most of the musculoskeletal structures are derived from undifferentiated mesoderm called mesenchyme. Differentiation of each portion of the mesenchyme is a continuous process, the outcome of which is not necessarily permanent, as the differentiated form expresses only part of the genetic material. Some stimulus is required to initiate the process of differentiation, which then usually persists without the stimulus.[2] Mechanical forces and movement have been identified as factors which alter musculoskeletal tissue structure during and after differentiation. Mechanical force and movement play a significant role in the postnatal development of the musculoskeletal structures and the strength of these structures, especially the organization of the fiber component, the amount of cross linkage of collagen, the size of the structure, the structure of junctions, and the development of joints.[3]

Cell shape, altered in vitro by mechanical forces, has been associated with changes in DNA synthesis, with an increase of DNA synthesis in flat cells and decrease of DNA synthesis in round cells.[4] As an example of a cellular property altered by mechanical forces, DNA synthesis can change the composition and strength of musculoskeletal structures. Although the possibility exists that voluntary and controlled application of force may be applied postnatally, application of this principle to the fetus usually involves naturally occurring forces, such as uterine constraint. An example of voluntarily applied force to the fetus would be external version or the manual force applied by the obstetrician attempting to change the position of the fetus in the uterus.

Specific loading conditions that may determine the effect of a force acting on a musculoskeletal structure include:

1. type of force–tensile (tending to separate), compressive (tending to crush), shear (tending to slide), bending (tending to curve), or torsion (tending to twist)
2. alignment or line of action and direction of the force
3. duration
4. frequency
5. intermittent or constant application
6. magnitude relative to tissue strength
7. rate of loading
8. pre-load tension of the tissue or structure
9. surface area distribution

Optimal mechanical forces are associated with normal development. Less than optimal or excessive mechanical forces can result in deformation.[5,6] Deformation resulting from mechanical forces is distinguished from malformation or disruption caused by genetic factors.[5] Mechanical forces can be internal or external to the person. Relevant external forces for the fetus include uterine characteristics, fetal numbers and positions, fetal to uterine contact forces, and buoyancy and drag (resistance to movement) of the amniotic fluid environment. For example, uterine constraint, in terms of diminished size or elasticity of the uterus, becomes an external force of potentially constraining magnitude after 20 weeks gestational age.[6]

External forces imposed on the fetus are different from the external forces imposed on the newborn infant. Buoyancy and drag of the amniotic fluid environment is replaced with a gravity environment, which involves a constant force pulling the body toward the earth's center. The newborn requires increased muscular force to initiate movement and once moving, experiences a greater tendency to keep moving (inertia). Fetal to uterine contact forces could occur with relatively equal frequency to any body part, as the uterus surrounds the fetus. Contact forces for the newborn usually involve body parts contacting external objects such as caretakers or firm surfaces, such as the floor.

Internal forces imposed on the fetus and the newborn are produced by muscle, tendon, ligament, bones, joint surfaces, and fascia. Examples of types of internal forces are:

1. tendon and ligament loads on bone causing tensile forces;
2. weight bearing on bones causing compressive forces, if the weight bearing is symmetrical and the bone is straight; bending forces, if the weight bearing is asymmetrical and/or the bone is bowed; and torsional forces, if the loads are of a twisting nature;
3. any bending or torsional force causing shear forces that tend to cause one structure to slide on another.

Changes in size and weight of total body or segmental proportions, locations of centers of mass, percentage and distribution of body fat, and the fluid versus gravity environment influence the effect of these external and internal forces on musculoskeletal development. In general, the genetic influence of development involves overall external shape of musculoskeletal structures, and the environmental influence of development affects discriminating aspects of shape and internal architecture. Both influences affect size in various dimensions. The effect of mechanical forces and movement on each musculoskeletal system structure will be discussed. A complete and sequential review of musculoskeletal development exists elsewhere.[7,8,9]

MUSCULOSKELETAL SYSTEM–COMPONENT STRUCTURES

Prenatal Limb Bone Development

Bone Formation. The limb bones traditionally have been thought to ossify by endochondral ossification, although growth of the limb bones may incorporate both membranous and endochondral ossification.[10,11] Bone formed by endochondral ossification is characterized by large changes in size during growth. Limb bones grow in length by growth plates and in width by the addition of cells from the perichondrium adjacent to hyaline cartilage, from specialized perichondrium called Zones of Ranvier at the periphery of the growth plate,[11] or from periosteum on the periphery of bone. After initial bone formation or modeling, compact bone in the shafts and outer areas, as well as trabecular bone in the ends or epiphyses and lining of the marrow cavities, are constantly being remodeled.

The general shape and most of the length of limb bones is genetically determined, whereas the bony prominences, width, angulation, and a small percentage of length are controlled by mechanical forces.[6] Frost[12] proposed that the effect of mechanical forces overrides the effect of genetic factors from the time of formation of the bony collar at eight weeks gestational age. Wolff's Law can be paraphrased to indicate the effect of mechanical forces on bone–where there is optimal stress (optimal loading conditions), bone deposition will be greater than bone resorption. Where there is nonoptimal stress related to inadequate or excessive loading conditions, bone resorption will be greater than bone deposition. Dynamic bending forces have a greater modeling/remodeling effect than compressive or tensile forces alone.[12] Growth plates align perpendicular or parallel to the primary force, usually compression or tension, on the plate. The plate aligns to minimize shear forces.[11,13] The plate is additionally protected from displacement caused by shear force by the formation of "hills and valleys," termed undulations and mammillary processes, respectively, and lateral projections toward the shaft, called lappet formations[11] (Figure 1). The effects of some mechanical forces on bones have not been distinguished specifically for the fetus. Table 1 includes the known effects of mechanical forces on prenatal skeletal development and on maturing bone. These effects have not been distinguished by age.

Skeletal Angles

Femur. Some prenatal skeletal angles change during normal development. The horizontal plane angle between the femoral neck and the distal femoral condyles (the angle of anteversion or neck-shaft torsional angle) changes dramatically from a retroverted position (posteriorly directed femoral head with respect to the axis of the femoral condyles) in the fetus to an anteverted position (anteriorly directed femoral head with respect to the axis of the femoral

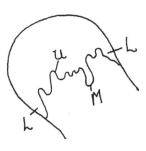

Figure 1. Fetal development of growth plates. Shown here is an epiphyseal plate, with undulations (U), mammillary processes (M), and lappet formations (L) in developing fetal bone. Adapted from Ogden, Grogan, and Light[11]

Table 1. Effect of Mechanical Forces on Prenatal Skeletal
Development

Force	Age	Effect of Force
Intermittent force-optimal loading conditions	Prior to maturity	Formation and maintenance of normal trabecular patterns[3,12]
		Increased bone cross section, density in bone[12]
		Cartilage formation in healing bone[3]
Intermittent compression with movement	Fetus	Development of articular cartilage[3]
-less than optimal loading conditions (i.e. loading with reduced magnitude)	Fetus	Bone resorption, decreased density[3,12]
-greater than optimal loading conditions (i.e. loading with excessive magnitude)	Fetus	Inhibited bone growth, greater resorption than deposition[3,12]
Constant load	Fetus	No effect or bone atrophy if the load is too great[3]
Immobilization	Fetus	Bone resorption[3,12]
	Fetus Child	Delayed secondary centers of ossification in the epiphyses of long bones if too little compression[14]
Compressive resultant force oriented nonperpendicular to epiphyseal plate	Before maturity	Realignment of the epiphyseal plate[3]

condyles) of 30-40° at birth compared to 8-15° in the adult.[15] The frontal plane angle made by the femoral neck and shaft (the angle of inclination)[16,17] has been reported to change less dramatically in angulation–from 175° in utero[16] compared to 120-135° in the adult.[15] The frontal plane tibiofemoral angle is in moderate genu varus at birth compared to the adult tibiofemoral angulation of 5-6° by 6 years old.[15,18,19, 20]

Tibia. The horizontal plane angulation between the proximal tibial condyles and the line between the medial and lateral malleoli (tibial torsion) is normally 5° of internal tibial torsion at birth compared to 15-30° of external tibial torsion in the adult.[21] The internal tibial torsion at birth probably is a result of uterine constraint, as medial tibial torsion does not occur in preterm infants.[22] Posterior slant of the tibial plateaus (retroversion) changes from a 27° slant at birth to a 5° slant at 19 years, while posterior bowing of the tibia (retroflexion) and posterior deflection of the tibia (retrotorsion) have not been observed at birth but occur postnatally.[16]

Foot. Four stages of prenatal foot development have been documented by Bohm and described by Tachijian.[20] In the first stage (8 weeks), the foot is characterized by about 90° of plantar flexion and marked adduction of the hindfoot and forefoot. In stage two (9 weeks), the foot is positioned in marked inversion and remains 90° plantar flexed. The metatarsals are adducted, the first metatarsal more than the others. In the third stage (10 weeks), plantar flexion decreases, but the inversion and metatarsal adduction of the second stage persist. In the fourth stage (12 weeks), the foot is less inverted and there is slight metatarsus varus. These stages reflect the reorientation of the talar neck from a medially tilted position of 35-75° in maximum inversion compared to the adult value of 12-32°. At birth the calcaneus is in 22° of varus alignment with the tibia, while the adult average alignment is 3° of varus.[20]

Forces on Limbs. Mechanical forces during prenatal development have not been well studied. Carter[14,23] successfully utilized assumed mechanical forces in the fetus in a finite element computer analysis to predict many aspects of prenatal skeletal development. The loading conditions, such as magnitude and duration, were established at arbitrary and equal values for an 8, 11 and 35 week fetus and were based on unknown internal muscular and external uterine forces as well as known femoral neck-shaft angles at different stages of embryonic and fetal development. Mechanical forces resulting from differential growth rates of limb structures appear to produce the rotation occurring within the humerus and femur in the eighth gestational week.[11]

Impairments of Limbs. Mechanical forces can affect the normal alteration of prenatal skeletal alignment. Retroversion or excessive anteversion may result from abnormal or constrained position of the fetus in the uterus. Constrained uterine position with the feet turned inward may result in excessive internal tibial torsion at birth, as well as such deformities as metatarsus adductus.[6] In the newborn who has paresis or paralysis during fetal development, the femur has a general characteristic shape, but is very slender with small trochanters and has a coxa valga of the femoral neck.[6] The coxa valga results from decreased muscular forces that would normally cause compression of the femoral head into the acetabulum (Figure 2). Muscular weakness of hip abductors and extensors, as a result of myelomeningocele, for example, may result in the abnormal angle of inclination of coxa valga (Figure 2).[12,21]

PRENATAL DEVELOPMENT

Muscles

By embryonic week eight, almost all skeletal muscles are present in the general shape of the adult muscle. Early muscular development, which includes both hyperplasia and hypertrophy,[25] is responsive to internal and external cues,[26] particularly tensile forces.[27] For the fetus, internal tensile forces result from muscular activation, and external tensile forces result from passive stretch due to uterine position or constraint. Specific loading conditions of these mechanical forces have not been well studied in prenatal development.

Tendons and Ligaments

Tendons and ligaments develop in situ directly from undifferentiated mesenchyme in the limbs.[28] The condensation of these structures can be observed in the 7th embryonic week.[28,29] Tendons

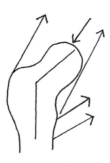 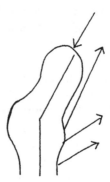

Fetal development with normal hip muscular forces

Fetal development with unbalanced hip muscular forces - here, with no hip abductors or extensors, as could occur with a lesion of the spinal cord at L3

Figure 2. Femoral neck-shaft angle in normal fetal growth and fetal growth with unbalanced muscular forces at the hip. This abnormal coxa valga angle of inclination could result from prenatal muscular weakness of the hip abductors and extensors resulting from myelomeningocele Adapted from 6,12,21,24

form parallel to the long axis of the muscle,[30] thus allowing the collagen fibers in tendon to be aligned to maximize their tensile strength properties. Tendon and ligament attachments remain a consistent relative distance from the joint surface by migration of the attachment site during growth. The migration occurs with sequential bony resorption and deposition around the attachment site.[11] Consistent shear forces on a localized area of tendon, appear to be the stimulus to form fibrocartilage at those contact sites. Examples of shear forces are the tendon-bone contact area of the obturator internus on the pelvis and the peroneus longus on the lateral malleolus. The mechanical properties of fibrocartilage allow this tissue to withstand shear forces better than tendon forces. The effects of forces on tendon and ligament before maturity have been determined postnatally, but they are included here because the effect could be the same on prenatal tendon and ligament (Table 2).

Junctions

Muscle-tendon junctions form prenatally as branches of split muscle fibers interdigitate with the collagen of tendon. The junction is not as interdigitated as in the adolescent or adult, and consequently, has less tensile strength in the fetus.[30]

Bones are joined to tendons and ligaments by junctions of transitional tissues that gradually reduce the potential stress concentration between the very stiff bone and the very flexible tendon or ligament. The transitional tissues, each sequentially stiffer than the last, are: the collagenous tendon or ligament, fibrocartilage, mineralized fibrocartilage, and bone.[34] Tensile loading at the junction sites appears to be the only mechanical stimulus required in formation of these tendon-bone and ligament-bone junctions.[3,26]

Table 2.   Effect of Mechanical Forces on Prenatal Development of Tendon and Ligament

Force	Age	Effect of force
Intermittent tension -optimal loading conditions	Before maturity	Increased tendon thickness and strength[24,31]
Intermittent tension -less than optimal loading conditions (eg loads of reduced magnitude)	Before maturity	Decreased tendon strength, stiffness and energy absorption[32,33]
Intermittent or constant tension- greater than optimal loading conditions (eg loads of excessive magnitude)	Before maturity	Failure by shearing of collagen fibers[33]
Constant tensile load	Before maturity	Tendon lengthening due to maintained tensile loading over a period of time[24]

Joints

Joint structures include the articular cartilage and the subchondral bone of two bone epiphyses; the joint capsule; intra-articular ligaments, tendons, or discs; synovial membrane; and synovial fluid. Interzone mesenchyme forms between the skeletal elements at the 5-6 week period.[7] Complete cavitation for human joints varies among joints but has been reported for human joints in general at 8 weeks[7] to 12 weeks.[35] Neither mechanical force nor movement seem required for initiation of human joint development or cavitation; however, movement at the joint site does appear necessary for complete cavitation.[29, 36] This movement may be caused by muscular activity and the mechanical effects of differential growth.[37] Many situations can affect the extent of fetal movement, e.g., too little amniotic fluid during late pregnancy is associated with decreased amplitude and speed of general fetal movements.[38]

The relationship between observable fetal joint movement and the formation of cavitation has yet to be established; however, fetal limb movements can be detected by ultrasound imaging at 8 weeks.[39,40,41,42] Further research will reveal the percent of cavitation required for observable fetal joint movement and the amount and type of joint movement required for complete cavitation and formation of normal joint surfaces.

Joint motion is determined by the bony congruity of the joint, shapes of the joint surfaces, angulation of skeletal elements, forces acting on the skeletal elements composing the joints, and structures guiding or limiting specific joint motions. Because of differential fetal growth rates of the acetabulum and femur, the hip joint has much better osseous congruity in early fetal development than in late fetal development.[43] This decreased congruity near birth facilitates passage of the fetus through the birth canal.[9] The congruity of the hip increases after birth as hip joint stability is required for optimal weight bearing.[6] Congruity increases as a result of muscular compressive forces, increased range of hip motion, and adequate positioning in hip abduction.

BIOMECHANICAL FACTORS DURING PRENATAL MOVEMENT

Joint movement occurs against opposing forces, some of which are quite different in the prenatal versus the postnatal environment.

Movement in the postnatal gravity environment is produced, maintained, or controlled by concentric, isometric, or eccentric muscle activations, respectively. Movement in the intrauterine fluid environment presumably involves concentric muscle activations, when acceleration occurs against the drag of the fluid medium, and eccentric or isometric muscle activations when deceleration or maintained postures, respectively, occurs in the presence of momentum of the fluid medium. Sparling et al.[44] have reported commonly observing fetal movement against the drag of the fluid medium followed by an apparent relaxation or floating of the body part back to the quiescent state. Biomechanical factors related to movement in a gravity environment are described in detail in Rodgers' work.[45]

The muscular requirement to produce a movement is increased if the effect of the resisting force is increased or the velocity of the movement is increased. In a gravity environment, increasing the magnitude of the resisting force and/or the moment arm of the resisting force will increase the muscular requirements to produce a specific movement. If movements occur against the pull of gravity, weights of specific segments of the body resist forces due to gravity. The location of the centers of mass is required to determine the moment arm for the segmental weight. Segmental proportions (size and weight of a body segment related to the body size) of the fetus are markedly different from those of the adult. The relatively large head and small arm, thigh, and calf of the fetus are the most striking differences compared to the adult.[7,18,46,47] Locations of centers of mass for each body segment have been reported for adults, especially adult white males.[48,49] Little is known about the center of mass locations for body segments in fetuses; however, the age-related body proportions result in a progressively inferior location of the body center of mass from the fetus to the adult. Body center of mass location has been documented at the thoracic 12 vertebral level for the 6 month-1 year old compared to the sacral 1 or 2 vertebral level for the adult.[15]

Location of the center of mass can be altered by changes in density within the segment, shape of the segment, and percentage and distribution of fat. Segmental density can be changed as structures within a segment mature, for example, as the hyaline cartilage models of the future long bones ossify from the shaft of the bone toward each bony end. In general, fetal limb segments could be geometrically modeled as cylinders,[50] whereas adult limb segments, except for the hand, would be more accurately modeled as truncated cones (cones with the pointed end removed),[51] because of the larger proximal end of the limb segment versus the smaller distal end. Percentage of body fat increases from 3.5 percent at 28 weeks to 7.5 percent at 34 weeks prenatally, continues to increase to 24 percent at 9 months-1 year postnatally, and decreases again from 5-7 years. These values can be compared to adult levels of 13-17 percent for men and 20-24 percent for women.[52]

ONGOING RESEARCH RELATED TO FETAL MOVEMENT

Current research in the Division of Physical Therapy at the University of North Carolina at Chapel Hill is aimed at validating a method of determining fetal limb segmental weights and centers of mass and quantifying knee angular velocities during fetal movement.

Fetal Limb Segmental Weights

The Hanavan method[51] of modeling the limb segments as geometrical shapes is being used to estimate fetal limb segmental weights by Riegger-Krugh, Schwarz, and Lawing (unpublished data, 1992). The fetuses are of varying ages and appear normal on visual observation. The arm, forearm, thigh, leg and foot are modeled as truncated cones, and the hand is modeled as a sphere. Proximal and distal segmental circumferences and segmental lengths are used to determine segmental volume, which is multiplied by an assumed limb density of 1.0 gm/cm^3 to determine the segmental mass. Segmental mass can be multiplied by the acceleration of gravity (9.8 m/sec) to determine segmental weight. The calculated segmental weight is compared to the direct weighing on a balance scale of the dissected segment to establish the validity of the method of determining segmental weight. Centers of mass for the segments are determined by balancing the dissected segment on a balance point and measuring the distance from the balance point to the proximal aspect of the segment.

From our observations, segmental weights for the thigh and foot are approximated by segmental weights calculated from the anthropometric measurements of circumference and segmental length. Altered operational definitions for anthropometric measurements of the arm, forearm, and leg may result in accurate approximation of segmental weight for those segments. Centers of mass for fetal limb segments appear centrally located in segments, whereas centers of mass for adult limb segments are located closer to the proximal joint of the segment[48,49] because of the proximal muscle bulk of the adult. Since the subjects are specimens who have died prenatally, the measured fetal segmental weights for a particular gestational age are not considered norms for that age.

Fetal movement can be observed by an ultrasound image. Fetal limb segmental weights have been determined using anthropometric measurements that may be obtainable from the ultrasound image.[54] If fetal limb segmental weights could be estimated from the fetal ultrasound image, norms could be established for segmental weight changes during specific prenatal ages. These norms are needed as one of many variables required to estimate the muscular forces during fetal movement. The specimens are normal appearing stillborn fetuses, as in the previous study. The hand, thigh, leg, and foot segmental weights can be accurately determined from these anthropometric measurements. Calculated arm and forearm segmental weights overestimate directly weighed segments. Altered operational definitions for arm and forearm segmental length are required here as in the previous study. Intra-rater and inter-rater reliability has been established for the anthropometric measurements in the range of .95-1.00 (Riegger-Krugh, Schwartz, Lawing, unpublished data, 1992). The validity of the anthropometric measurements obtained from the ultrasound image as compared to actual measurements in the fetus must be established before this method can be used to estimate fetal segmental weight in vivo.

Fetal Knee Joint Angular Velocity

In a third study, a method for measuring fetal knee joint angular velocity has been established.[54] Joint movement characteristics, such as angular velocity, are important aspects of normal fetal movement strategies and may prove useful in early detection of fetal distress or pathology. Fetal movement has been qualitatively assessed[39,44] and quantitatively assessed relative to frequency and duration of fetal movement,[40] but angular joint motion has not been measured previously in the fetus. In our study, ultrasound images of the fetal lower limb taken perpendicular to the ultrasound head were measured by placing a goniometer on the TV monitor screen. A training procedure was established to obtain reliability of two testers, who measured knee joint angular velocity. The ranges of angular velocity that correspond to qualitative intervals of knee velocity–slow, moderately slow, moderate, moderately fast, and fast–have been incorporated into the Force Quality portion of a fetal movement assessment (Q-Move) developed by Green and Sparling[44] and described in this issue.

CONCLUSIONS

The effects of mechanical forces and movement on prenatal development of the musculoskeletal system have been reviewed. Physical and occupational therapists use both factors as a basis for their patient evaluation and treatment intervention. Knowledge of the effects of these factors should enhance understanding of the biomechanical basis of normal and abnormal prenatal musculoskeletal development and stimulate research questions related to the application of these factors to fetuses.

REFERENCES

1. VanSant A. A lifespan development of functional tasks. *Phys Ther.* 1990; 70:788-798.

2. Buckwalter JA, Cooper RR. The cells and matrices of the skeletal connective tissues. In: Albright JA, Brand RA, eds. *The Scientific Basis of Orthopaedics*, 2nd Ed. Norwalk, CT: Appleton and Lange; 1987, pp 1-29.

3. Storey E. Growth and remodeling of bone and bones. *Dental Clin NA.* 1975;19(3):443-455.

4. Folkman J, Moscona A. Role of cell shape in growth control. *Nature.* 1978;273:345-349.

5. Dunne KB, Clarren SK. The origin of prenatal and postnatal deformities. *Ped Clin of N.A.* 1986;33(6):1277-1297.

6. Smith DW. *Recognizable Patterns of Human Deformity: Identification and Management of Mechanical Effects on Morphogenesis.* Philadelphia:WB Saunders Co; 1981.

7. Moore KL. *Before We Were Born.* 3rd ed. Philadelphia: WB Saunders Co; 1989.

8. Sadler TW. *Langman's Medical Embryology.* Baltimore: Williams and Wilkins Co;1985.

9. Walker JM. Musculoskeletal development: a review. *Phys Ther.* 1991; 71:878-889.

10. Ogden JA, Grogan DP: Prenatal development and growth of the musculoskeletal system. In: Albright JA, Brand RA, eds. *The Scientific Basis of Orthopaedics,* 2nd ed. Norwalk, CT: Appleton and Lange; 1987, pp 47-89.

11. Ogden JA, Grogan DP, Light TR: Postnatal development and growth of the musculoskeletal system. In: Albright JA, Brand RA, eds. *The Scientific Basis of Orthopaedics,* 2nd ed. Norwalk, CT: Appleton and Lange; 1987, pp 91-160.

12. Frost HM: Mechanical determinants of skeletal architecture: Bone modeling. In: Albright JA, Brand RA, eds. *The Scientific Basis of Orthopaedics,* 2nd ed. Norwalk, CT: Appleton and Lange; 1987, pp 241-265.

13. Smith JW. The relationship of epiphyseal plates to stress in some bones of the lower limb. *J Anat.* 1962;96:58-80.

14. Carter DR, Orr TE, Fyhrie DP, Schurman DJ. Influences of mechanical stress on prenatal and postnatal skeletal development. *Clin Orth Rel Res.* 1987; 219:237-250.

15. Magee DJ. *Orthopedic Physical Assessment.* Philadelphia: WB Saunders Co; 1987.

16. Bernhardt D. Prenatal and postnatal growth and development of the foot and ankle. *Phys Ther.* 1988;68:1831-1839.

17. Soderberg GL. *Kinesiology: Application to Pathological Motion.* Baltimore: Williams and Wilkins Co;1986.

18. Salenius P, Vankka E. The development of the tibiofemoral angle in children. *J Bone Jt Surg.* 1975;57-A(2):259-261.

19. Tachdjian MO. *Pediatric Orthopedics.* Philadelphia:WB Saunders Co; 1972.

20. Tachdjian MO. *The Child's Foot.* Philadelphia: WB Saunders Co;1985.

21. Bunch W. Origin and mechanism of postnatal deformities. *Ped Clin of NA.* 1977;24(4):679-684.

22. Katz K, Naor N, Merlob, and Wielunsky E. Rotational deformities of the tibia and foot in preterm infants. *J Ped Orth.* 1990;10:483-485.

23. Carter DR, Wong M. Mechanical stresses in joint morphogenesis and maintenance. In: Mow VC, Ratcliffe A, Woo SLY, eds. *Biomechanics of Diarthrodial Joints,* Vol II., New York: Springer-Verlag;1990, pp 155-174.

24. Frost H. *The Physiology of Cartilaginous, Fibrous, and Bony Tissue.* Orthopedic Lectures. Springfield, IL: Charles C Thomas; 1972.

25. Mastaglia FL. Growth and development of skeletal muscle. In: Davis JA, Dobbing J, eds. *Scientific Foundations of Paediatrics*. Baltimore, MD: University Park Press; 590-620, 1981.

26. Woo SLY, Buckwalter JA, eds. *Injury and Repair of Musculoskeletal Soft Tissues*. Park Ridge, IL: American Academy of Orthopaedic Surgeons; 1987.

27. Tickle C, Wopert L. Limb Development. In: Davis JA, Dobbing J, eds. *Scientific Foundations of Paediatrics*. Baltimore, MD: University Park Press; 1981, pp 544-564.

28. O'Railly R, Gardner E. The timing and sequence of events in the development of the limbs in the human embryo. *Anat Embryol*. 1975;148:1-23.

29. O'Railly R, Gardner E. The embryology of movable joints. In: Sokoloff L, ed. *The Joints and Synovial Fluid*. Vol I. New York: Academic Press; 1978, pp 49-103.

30. Ovalle WK. The human muscle-tendon junction. *Anat Embryol*. 1987;176: 281-294.

31. Cornwall M, LeVeau BF. The effect of physical activity on ligamentous strength: an overview. *J Orth Sport Phys Ther*. 1984;5:275-277.

32. Tipton CM, Matthes RD, Maynard JA, Carey JA. The influence of physical activity on ligaments and tendons. *Med Sci Sports*. 1976;7:165-175.

33. Noyes F, Trovik P, Hyde W, DeLucas JL. Biomechanics of ligament failure. II. An analysis of immobilization, exercise, and reconditioning effects in primates. *J Bone Joint Surg*. 1974;56A:1406-1418.

34. Cooper RR, Misol S. Tendon and ligament insertion. *J Bone Joint Surg*. 1970;52A:1-21.

35. Crelin ES. *Clinical Symposium: Development of the Musculoskeletal System*. 33(1). Summit, NJ: Ciba Pharmaceutical Co; 1981.

36. Drachman DB, Sokoloff L. The role of movement in embryonic joint development. *Develop Biol*. 1966;14:401-420.

37. Fell HB, Canti RG. Experiments on the development in vitro of the avian knee joint. *Proc R Soc London*. 1934;Ser. B 116:316-351.

38. Sival DA, Visser GHA, Prechtl HFR. Does reduction of amniotic fluid affect fetal movements? *Early Hum Dev*. 1990;23:233-246.

39. deVries JIP, Visser GHA, Prechtl HFR. The emergence of fetal behavior I. Qualitative aspects. *Early Hum Dev*. 1982;7:301-322.

40. deVries JIP, Visser GHA, Prechtl HFR. The emergence of fetal behavior II. Quantitative aspects. *Early Hum Dev*. 1985;12:99-120.

41. deVries JIP, Visser GHA, Prechtl HFR. The emergence of fetal behavior III. Individual differences and consistencies. *Early Hum Dev*. 1988;16:85-103.

42. Ianniruberto A, Tajani E. Ultrasonographic study of fetal movements. *Semin Perinatol*. 1981;5:175-181.

43. Walker JM, Goldsmith CH. Morphometric study of the fetal development of the human hip joint: significance for congenital hip disease. *Yale J Biol Med*. 1981;54:411-437.

44. Sparling JW, Wilhelm IJ, McLeod AM, Green S, Katz V, Blanchard G, et al. Developing a taxonomy of fetal movement: The first step in a longitudinal collaborative study. *Phys Occup Ther Pediatri*. 1990;10(1):43-46.

45. Rodgers MM. Musculoskeletal considerations in production and control of movement. In: Montgomery PC, Connolly BH, eds. *Motor Control and Physical Therapy: Theoretical Framework and Practical Applications.* 1st ed. Chattanooga, TN: Chattanooga Group, Inc.; 1991, pp 47-61.

46. Jensen RK. Body segment mass, radius, and radius of gyration proportions in children. *J Biomech.* 1986;19(5):359-368.

47. Scammon RE, Calkins LA. *Growth in the Fetal Period.* Minneapolis: The University of Minnesota Press; 1929.

48. Clauser CE, McConville JT, Young JW. Weight, Volume, and Center of Mass Segments of the Human Body. Ohio: Wright-Patterson Air Force Base, (AMRL-TR-69-70); 1969.

49. Dempster WT. Space requirements of the seated operator. Ohio: Wright-Patterson Air Force Base (WADCTR 55-159); 1955.

50. Picker R, Saunders D. A simple geometrical method for determining fetal weight in utero with compound gray scale ultrasound scan. *Am J Obstet Gyn.* 1976;124:493-494.

51. Hanavan EP. A mathematical model of the human body. Ohio: Wright-Patterson Air Force Base (AMRL Technical Report 64-102); 1964.

52. Davis JA, Dobbing J, ed. *Scientific Foundations of Paediatrics.* Philadelphia: WB Saunders Co; 1974.

53. Riegger-Krugh C. Determination of fetal limb segmental weights using anthropometric measurements. *Phys Ther.* 1991;71:S95.

54. Riegger-Krugh C, Blair A, Sparling JW. Qualitative and quantitative assessment of knee angular velocity in fetal movement. Presented at the North Carolina Physical Therapy Association Conference. Asheville, NC: October 22-25, 1992.

The Origins
of the Mother-Child Relationship–
A Review

Mecca S. Cranley

SUMMARY. Evidence is mounting that the relationship of a woman with her child is initiated during pregnancy as the woman begins to develop her maternal role. The nature of this beginning relationship, referred to as maternal attachment to the fetus, is reviewed together with the research into factors which enhance or impede it. Evidence for the continuum of attachment through gestation into the postnatal period is considered and issues of reliability and validity are raised. Areas for further research and the clinical urgency of discovering successful interventions are discussed.

The relationship of mother and child may be both the most heralded and the most condemned of all human relationships. It has inspired sublime paintings and poetry as well as vitriolic exposés of lives ruined by supposed maternal fault. Without doubt it is a relationship, at least in its beginnings, of unparalleled power imbalance. The infant in total dependency relies on the good will of the mother to provide first life itself, then nourishment, shelter and safety. But that is not all. Harlow, Harlow and Hansen,[1] working with Rhesus monkeys, and Bowlby,[2,3] working with human children, provided striking evidence that meeting the child's physiological needs, while necessary, is not sufficient for healthy social and psychological development. In Harlow's terms, what is required is "mother love"; Bowlby labeled it "attachment."

Mecca S. Cranley, RN, PhD, is Dean and Professor at the School of Nursing, State University of New York at Buffalo.

How does mother love come about? When does attachment begin? This paper will explore the evidence available in the literature that the emotional investment in and relationship with her child begins during a woman's pregnancy.

THE BEGINNING OF ATTACHMENT

Pregnancy as a developmental stage has been described by Deutsch,[4] Benedek,[5-7] and Bibring.[8] Erikson, in discussing the stage of Generativity versus Stagnation, gave a general overview of the tasks of pregnancy when he described a "gradual expansion of ego-interest and . . . a libidinal investment in that which is being generated."[9,p267] Deutsch,[4] Tanner,[10] and Rubin[11] more specifically described a progression of investing the fetus with narcissistic love, then gradually differentiating the fetus from herself and increasingly appreciating a separate individual. Tanner related these stages to the physical events of pregnancy, particularly quickening and subsequent fetal activity. Rubin identified four developmental tasks of pregnancy and, using analysis of detailed case information, described how women behave while working on each of these tasks during the three trimesters of gestation. In sum, there is consensus in this literature that while the fetus is developing physically during pregnancy, there occurs simultaneously an equally dynamic development of the woman into a mother.

Despite this consensus, the predominant viewpoint prior to 1980 was that the relationship or attachment between mother and child begins with birth and progresses rapidly during the early postpartum period. From the mid 1970's the lay public and health professionals alike had been captivated by the now famous studies of Klaus and Kennell[12] who described a "critical period" just after birth when mothers, and perhaps infants, were best suited to "bond" with each other. Although these studies were responsible for bringing about much needed reform in hospital maternity care, the concept of the critical period adapted from animal studies has failed to hold up in repeated studies. Moreover, this postnatal beginning of attachment appears inconsistent with women's experiences of pregnancy. Thus the 1980's saw the development of exploration into the alternative hypothesis that women in fact begin to develop their relationships with their children during the prenatal period and the term maternal-fetal attachment was coined.[13]

THE NATURE OF THE PRENATAL RELATIONSHIP

Although early descriptions of the woman's relationship with her unborn child had their origins in psychoanalytic theory and were primarily the result of observations of pregnant women in therapy, several descriptive studies were conducted. Rubin[11] identified "bind-ing in to the fetus" as one of four developmental tasks to be accomplished by the pregnant woman in preparation for giving birth. She described this as an acquaintance process through which the woman comes to know, have affection for and interact with the fetus as a separate individual. Rubin saw the binding in process as a continuum which extended through birth into the postpartum period. Muller[14] has reviewed three descriptive studies by Leifer,[15] Lumley,[16,17] and Stainton.[18] Interviewing relatively small samples of women (19, 30 and 25, respectively), these researchers all reported that the women described interaction and communication with their unborn children. They ascribed individual characteristics to them and reported feelings of love.

Cranley[13] developed the Maternal-Fetal Attachment Scale (MFA) to attempt to measure the concept of a mother's relationship to her fetus prior to birth. Both in the development and in the utilization of that scale in research, women have responded with enthusiasm to items that indicate feelings of affiliation and affection toward their unborn children. Research subjects who complete the scale frequently express delight at items indicating that they speak or sing to the fetus, give it a pet name, do things to insure its health, attribute intentions to it or have fantasies about their life together. Thus a convincing body of literature supports the concept of mothers' developing attachment to their children during their pregnancies. Multiple studies utilizing the Cranley MFA have been reported. Condon,[19,20] using the term "antenatal attachment" and a scale which he developed that is similar to the MFA, reported findings for expectant mothers and fathers that are very similar to those reported by investigators using the MFA.

In summary, although ample evidence exists that women do, indeed, have relationships with the fetuses that they nurture through nine months of gestation, how that relationship develops and what circumstances trigger, stimulate or stifle it is the subject of considerable interest and investigation in social science and health care literature. As the birth rate has declined in Western societies and the conceptions of marriage and the family have undergone marked change, the task of identifying early predictors of healthy parent-child relationships has achieved prominence.[21] Research during the past decade has focused on the correlates of maternal-fetal attachment (both positive and negative) and on the association between prenatal attachment and the parent-infant relationship after birth.

CORRELATES OF MATERNAL-FETAL ATTACHMENT

Personal and situational variables have been examined in association with prenatal attachment in an effort to discover factors which may influence its development. Presumably these findings would be expected to lead ultimately to the articulation of preventive and therapeutic intervention strategies. Of the many variables associated with prenatal attachment in various studies, four have had consistent correlations over more than one study. These four are quickening, gestational age, risk status and marital relationship. Quickening and gestational age correlate positively with maternal-fetal attachment scores.[15-17,21-26] Marital satisfaction has also consistently been found to be positively associated with maternal-fetal attachment.[27-29] Gloger-Tippelt,[21] although not measuring marital satisfaction as such, found a strong positive relationship between the mother's prenatal conceptions of her fetus and the duration of the marital partnership. Lindner[30] reported that for single, pregnant adolescents there was a significant correlation between maternal-fetal attachment and the presence of a current, emotionally close relationship with the infant's father. Pregnancy risk status has also been consistent in not being correlated at all with prenatal attachment.[28,31,32]

In a 1992 review of much of the research in which the Cranley Maternal-Fetal Attachment Scale has been used, Muller has discussed the disparate findings with regard to the following variables: demographic factors (age, socioeconomic status, race, number of children, education), social support, anxiety, ultrasound visualization of the fetus and amniocentesis. With respect to demography, social support and anxiety, various researchers have found positive, negative and no correlations for these variables. For an excellent review and table of these studies, the reader is referred to the Muller publication.

Several clinical investigators[33-35] have described an increase in women's awareness and regard for the fetus after experiencing ultrasound visualization. Heidrich and Cranley,[23] in a quasi-experimental study with a control group of women not having an ultrasound, reported that ultrasound scanning had no effect on maternal-fetal attachment. Gloger-Tippelt,[21] using a cognitive model in a cross-sectional, descriptive study, found that the more women had a clear ultrasound picture of the fetus, the more they regarded the child as an independent human being and as an individual person. Attachment and cognitive awareness of the fetus as an independent person, however, may be different variables, which may not be mutually exclusive. In future studies of the effects of ultrasound, investigating the effects of ultrasound scanning at different gestational ages would be helpful. Reported positive effects may be explained by the developmental characteristics of the women's attitudes toward the fetus as pregnancy progresses.

Although most investigators of maternal-fetal attachment have attempted to explicate the factors that are positively associated with this attachment, several studies have been reported in which variables were identified that have a negative effect. Lindner[30] studied 67 pregnant adolescent girls, 33 of whom were planning to place their babies for adoption and 34 of whom were planning to keep them. Those who were planning to place the babies for adoption scored significantly lower on the MFA Scale than the keeping group. It cannot be determined from the data whether these young women decided to place their babies for adoption because they were not attached to them or withheld their attachment to protect themselves from the hurt of impending separation. In a study of surrogate motherhood, Fischer and Gillman[36] found the 21 surrogate mothers to be significantly less attached to the fetus than the 21 mothers in the comparison group. Women who undergo amniocentesis for genetic diagnosis have been described as withholding attachment until reassuring results are obtained.[32,37-39] Condon,[40] writing in the psychiatric literature about fetal abuse, includes low attachment to the fetus as his first risk factor for this behavior. Condon and Hilton[41] further report that increased feelings of attachment are predictive of a decrease or even cessation of alcohol consumption during pregnancy but not of cigarette smoking.

RELATIONSHIP TO POSTNATAL ATTACHMENT

Maternal-fetal attachment has been conceptualized as part of a continuum of attachment which begins during pregnancy and extends into the postnatal relationship of mother and child.[13,42] Although this concept is intuitively satisfying, attempts to demonstrate it empirically have been less than successful. Leifer[15] reported that a woman's psychological functioning early in pregnancy predicted both her attachment to the fetus and to the infant after birth. Cranley[13,42] identified a modest correlation between maternal-fetal attachment and the woman's score on a subset of items about "average" babies from the Neonatal Perception Inventory. Reading et al.[25] reported a positive relationship between attachment at 32 weeks gestation and at 24 hours after birth but the relationship no longer existed at 3 months after birth. Fuller,[43] in a master's thesis, investigated 32 women, and reported a significant correlation between the scores on the MFA Scale at 35 to 40 weeks gestation and scores on the Nursing Child Assessment Feeding Scale (NCAFS).[44] To date, however, that study has not been published nor has it been replicated. In a study of the relationship between prenatal attachment and parents' later perception of their infants' temperaments, Wolk,[45] measured attachment to the fetus at 32-33 weeks gestation in 44 couples. Attachment scores contributed significantly to the explanation of variance in perceptions of infant temperament at three months of age.

Efforts to confirm any progression of attachment through pregnancy, its effect on the birth experience and its continuation into postnatal attachment have been hindered by a lack of longitudinal studies. Those longitudinal studies which have been reported either have been limited to pregnancy itself[22,24] or have continued data collection only into the first few days postpartum. Although Wolk et al.[45] followed the subjects for as long as three months, they were investigating the effect of parents' attachment to the fetus on their perceptions of infant temperament, not the continuum of attachment as such. The lack of a postnatal attachment instrument with demonstrated reliability and validity across studies is another obstacle in determining the relationship between pre- and postnatal attachment.

THREATS TO VALIDITY OF RESEARCH

An advantage in evaluating the research on maternal-fetal attachment is that the majority of investigators have used one instrument to measure attachment. A disadvantage is that, to the extent that the instrument is flawed, the multiple studies continue to perpetuate the same errors. Other variables, even when they have the same name across several studies, have seldom been measured by the same instruments. Thus it is difficult to compare several studies in which social support has been investigated, for example, when each study has used a different measure of social support. For a comprehensive discussion of issues of validity, see Muller[14] and Cranley.[46]

Given the relative newness of the field of study in this area as well as the lack of a consistently emerging explanatory model, it is not surprising that very little intervention research has been done. Most intervention researchers have taken advantage of already occurring medical treatments such as ultrasound or amniocentesis. Only Heidrich and Cranley[23] have reported a study with both pre- and post-tests of the subjects and a comparison group that did not receive the treatment.

Two studies have been reported in which fetal activity was used as the variable that was related to fetal attachment. Zeanah et al.[47] investigated 44 couples each expecting their first child. Objective measures of fetal activity were obtained during each of two sonograms and by parents counting fetal movements using a stop watch.

Parents were also asked for a subjective description of fetal activity during routine situations. Both mothers and fathers who reported more intense feelings of attachment to their fetuses perceived them to be more active. Mikhail et al.[48] used an experimental design to examine the effect of fetal movement counting on maternal-fetal attachment. Subjects were 213 women who were randomly assigned to one of three groups: either a control group or one of two treatment groups who were instructed to count fetal movements according to two different methods recommended in the obstetric literature for such counting. All women completed the MFA Scale prior to beginning the study and again after one month. Women in both treatment groups scored significantly higher on the MFA than did the women in the control group who did not count fetal movements. This study is of further interest because more than two-thirds of the subjects were either African-American or Hispanic, unmarried and unemployed. This contrasts with the majority of studies of maternal-fetal attachment which have included subjects who were predominantly white, middle class and relatively well educated.

FUTURE DIRECTIONS

To date, no single explanatory model has consistently emerged from the research to structure thinking or guide interventions to promote attachment between pregnant women and the fetuses they carry. Yet an urgency exists to illuminate the mechanisms of maternal role development for at least two reasons: to reassure those parents who are struggling to do everything "right" and to motivate those parents, especially those mothers, who are unaware or unconcerned about their own impact on their developing fetus.

The imagination of the middle class public has been captured by books in the mall bookstores such as *The Life Within*,[49] and *The Tentative Pregnancy*.[39] The syndicated comic strip, Cathy, contained multiple episodes during which Cathy's pregnant friend played Mozart, spoke French and recited poetry to her fetus in an attempt to develop a superior child. These materials offer opportunity for expectant parents to learn and grow, but also set up performance standards that may be unrealistic for the best of parents. For example, Verny and Kelly write: "Whether his mind evolves into something essentially hard, angular and dangerous or soft, flowing and open depends largely on whether [the mother's] thoughts and emotions are positive and reinforcing or negative and etched with ambivalence."[49,p29] Who can live, never mind being pregnant, for nine months without any negative or ambivalent thoughts and feelings?

On the other hand, some women appear to lack the ability to care enough to provide a safe intrauterine environment for their children. These women give birth to a frightening number of newborn infants who must bear the burden of life-long physical and intellectual handicaps resulting from alcohol, cocaine and other drug abuse, preterm birth and low birth weight. If intervention exists which can instill, teach or foster different maternal behaviors because of an attachment to the child, such interventions must be found before a generation is wasted.

In Western society, conceptions of marriage and the family have undergone drastic modifications in recent years. Until society accommodates to these changes, it will be less likely that there will be a naturally occurring safety net of a larger family and community to help the parent help the child. Increasing numbers of children will spend a portion of their childhood living in a single parent household where the adults frequently are stressed by poverty, lack of a supportive network and the hopelessness that comes from a paucity of life options. Many children live in complex and frequently changing families that require them to adapt to a series of step-parents and step-siblings, shifting custody arrangements and confusing emotions. These events place a burden on the helping professions to discover early clues to an individual's likelihood of successful parenting and interventions to develop or enhance that likelihood.

To date, the research on women's relationships with their unborn infants has been guided by the paradigm of attachment, a paradigm developed initially to explain an infant's relationship with his/her caregiver and only later extended to include the mother in a transactional model. The further extension of attachment into time beyond the first two years of life poses many interesting questions for the researcher. For instance, the manifestations of attachment seem likely to change over time as the relationship matures and as the child is born and grows older and capable of entering into much more complex interactions. In other words, is attachment the same between parents and infants as between parents and six-year-olds or parents and adolescents? How is the attachment between parents and their adult children affected by aging parents who may be cared for by their children? These are interesting questions to unravel, but because of the practical urgency for the helping professions to find ways to help parents, it may be more fruitful to shift our attention from the model provided by attachment theory.

Two other approaches may be helpful. Because the clinician's goal often is to identify individuals who are at risk to be unsuccessful parents, and to prevent unsuccessful parenting from occurring by eliminating or reducing the risk factor(s), it may be profitable to couch the problem in a risk assessment framework. Alternatively, if the goal is to understand why women do or do not form affectional bonds with their fetuses, it may be helpful to consider a cognitive model. Bretherton[50] has discussed the importance of a woman elaborating an "internal working model" of her child and herself-as-parent. Gloger-Tippelt[51] has described the cognitive processes by which the parent develops a cognition of the fetus during pregnancy. Consideration of these paradigms, and others, may broaden the investigation into parents' relationships with their unborn infants, suggest new variables to investigate, new methodologies to employ and produce new and richer outcomes. Our children may depend on it.

REFERENCES

1. Harlow H, Harlow M, Hansen E. The maternal affectional system of rhesus monkeys. In: Rheingold HL, ed. *Maternal Behavior in Mammals.* New York: Wiley; 1963:254-281.

2. Bowlby J. The nature of the child's tie to his mother. *Int J Psychoanal.* 1958;39:350-373.

3. Bowlby J. *Attachment and Loss*, Vol. 1, *Attachment.* London: Hogarth Press; 1969.

4. Deutsch H. *Psychology of Women*, Vol. II. New York: Grune and Stratton; 1945.

5. Benedek T. The psycho-somatic implications of the primary unit. *Am J Orthopsychiatry.* 1949;19:642-654.

6. Benedek T. Parenthood as a developmental phase. *J Am Psychoanal Assoc.* 1959;7:389-417.

7. Benedek T. The psychobiology of pregnancy. In: Anthony EJ, Benedek T, eds. *Parenthood, Its Psychology and Psychopathology.* New York: Little, Brown; 1970, pp137-151.

8. Bibring GL. A study of the psychological processes in pregnancy and of the earliest mother-child relationship. *Psychoanal Study Child.* 1959;14:113-121.

9. Erikson EH. *Childhood and Society.* New York: W.W. Norton; 1950.

10. Tanner LM. Developmental tasks of pregnancy. In: Bergersen BS, et al, eds. *Current Concepts in Clinical Nursing,* Vol. II. St. Louis, MO: Mosby; 1969:292-297.

11. Rubin R. Maternal tasks in pregnancy. *Mat Child Nurs J.* 1975;4:143-153.

12. Klaus MH, Kennell JH. Mothers separated from their newborn infants. *Ped Clin North Am.* 1970;17:1015-1037.

13. Cranley M. Development of a tool for the measurement of maternal attachment during pregnancy. *Nurs Res.* 1981;30:281-284.

14. Muller M. A critical review of prenatal attachment research. *Sch Inq Nurs.* 1992;6(1):5-22.

15. Leifer M. Psychological changes accompanying pregnancy and motherhood. *Genet Psychol Monogr.* 1977;95:55-96.

16. Lumley J. The image of the fetus in the first trimester. *Birth Fam J.* 1980;2(1):5-14.

17. Lumley J. Attitudes to the fetus among primigravidae. *Aust Paediatr J.* 1982;18:106-109.

18. Stainton M. The fetus: A growing member of the family. *Fam Relat.* 1985;34:321-326.

19. Condon J. The parental-foetal relationship–a comparison of male and female expectant parents. *J Psychosom Obstet Gynecol.* 1985;4:271-284.

20. Condon J. Nature and determinants of parent to infant attachment in the early postnatal period. *J Am Acad Child Psych.* 1988;27(3):293-299.

21. Gloger-Tippelt G. The development of the mother's conceptions of the child before birth. Paper presented at the Sixth Biennial International Conference on Infant Studies. Washington, DC; 1988.

22. Grace J. Development of maternal-fetal attachment during pregnancy. *Nurs Res.* 1989;38(4):228-232.

23. Heidrich S. Cranley M. Effect of fetal movement, ultrasound scans and amniocentesis on maternal-fetal attachment. *Nurs Res.* 1989;38(2):81-84.

24. LoBiondo-Wood G. The progression of physical symptoms in pregnancy and the development of maternal-fetal attachment. Rochester, NY: University of Rochester; 1985. Dissertation.

25. Reading A, Cox D, Sledmere C, Campbell S. Psychological changes over the course of pregnancy: a study of attitudes toward the fetus/neonate. *Health Psychol.* 1984;3:211-221.

26. Vito KO. The development of maternal-fetal attachment and the association of selected variables. *Dissertation Abstracts International.* 47:998-B; 1986.

27. Cranley M. Social support as a factor in the development of parents' attachment to their unborn. *Birth Defects*. 1984;20:99-109.

28. Mercer R, Ferketich S, May K, DeJoseph J, Sollid D. Further exploration of maternal- and paternal-fetal attachment. *Res Nurs Health*. 1988;11:83-95.

29. Weaver R, Cranley M. An exploration of paternal fetal attachment behavior. *Nurs Res*. 1983;33:229-234.

30. Lindner EA. Maternal-fetal attachment in the pregnant adolescent, self-esteem, relationship with mother, and the decision to keep or release the infant for adoption. Madison, WI: University of Wisconsin-Madison;1984. Dissertation.

31. Curry MS. Maternal behavior of hospitalized pregnant women. *J Psychosomat Obstet Gynecol*. 1987;7:165-182.

32. Kemp VH, Page CK. Maternal prenatal attachment in normal and high-risk pregnancies. *J Obstet Gynecol Neonatal Nurs*. 1987;16:179-184.

33. Fletcher J, Evans M. Maternal bonding in early fetal ultrasound examination. *New Eng J Med*. 1983;308:392-393.

34. Kohn CL, Nelson A, Weiner S. Gravida's responses to realtime ultrasound fetal image. *J Obstet Gyecol Neonatl Nurs*. 1980;9:77-80.

35. Milne L, Rich O. Cognitive and affective aspects of the responses of pregnant women to sonography. *Mat Child Nurs J*. 1981;10:15-39.

36. Fischer S, Gillman I. Surrogate motherhood: attachment, attitudes and social support. *Psychiatry*. 1991;54: 13-20.

37. Phipps S, Zinn A. Psychological response to amniocentesis: I. mood state and adaptation to pregnancy. *Am J Med Genet*. 1986;25:131-142.

38. Phipps S, Zinn A. Psychological response to amniocentesis: II. effects of coping style. *Am J Med Genet*. 1986;25:143-148.

39. Rothman BK. The Tentative Pregnancy: *Prenatal Diagnosis and the Future of Motherhood*. New York: Penguin Books; 1987.

40. Condon J. The spectrum of fetal abuse in pregnant women. *J Nervous Mental Disease*. 1986;174(9):509-516.

41. Condon J, Hilton CA. Comparison of smoking and drinking behaviors in pregnant women: who abstains and why. *Med J Aust*. 1988;148:381-385.

42. Cranley M. Roots of attachment: The relationship of parents with their unborn. *Birth Defects*. 1981;17(6), 59-83.

43. Fuller J. The development of maternal attachment from fetal affiliation to infant interaction. Halifax, Nova Scotia, Canada: Dalhousie University; 1984.

44. Barnard K. *Nursing Child Assessment Feeding Scales*. Seattle, WA: University of Washington; 1978.

45. Wolk S, Zeanah CH, Coll CTG, Carr S. Factors affecting parents perceptions of temperament in early infancy. *Am J Orthopsych*. 1992;62(1):71-82.

46. Cranley M. Response to a critical review of prenatal attachment research. *Sch Inq Nurs*. 1992;6(1):23-26.

47. Zeanah C, Carr S, Wolk S. Fetal movements and the imagined baby of pregnancy: are they related? *J Reprod Infant Psychol*. 1990;8:23-36.

48. Mikhail M, Freda M, Merkatz R, Rolizzotto R, Mazloom E, Merkatz I. The effect of fetal movement counting on maternal attachment to fetus. *Am J Obstet.Gynecol.* 1991;165:988-991.

49. Verny T, Kelly J. *The Secret Life of the Unborn Child.* New York: Dell Publishing; 1981.

50. Bretherton J. Attachment theory: retrospect and prospect. In: Bretherton J, Waters E, eds. *Growing point of attachment. Monographs of the Society for Research in Child Development.* 1985;50(209):3-39.

51. Gloger-Tippelt G. A process model of the pregnancy course. *Hum Dev.* 1983;26:134-148.

Obstetric Ultrasound:
An Overview

Vern L. Katz

SUMMARY. Uses of ultrasound are expanding to include a variety of diagnostic activities ranging from evaluating detailed anatomy, to identifying at-risk fetuses, to assessing uterine insufficiency. Because of these uses, ultrasound is a necessary component of prenatal care and research related to fetal and maternal health. This paper deals on a basic level with how ultrasound is used in obstetrics.

INTRODUCTION

In the past generation the use of ultrasound has revolutionized the practice of obstetrics. The visualization and assessment of the fetus within the uterus has helped clinicians and researchers to answer questions about the physiology of pregnancy, about embryology, and to catalogue normal and abnormal development. Because ultrasound is painless and noninvasive, it has been widely adopted into the obstetricians' practice. As a result, most parents are now able to see their babies prior to birth. The psychological changes resulting from this visualization potentially have modified bonding patterns developed over thousands of years. Incredibly, these changes have occurred within a span of a single generation. In addition, the physician's approach to the patient has been altered by

Vern L. Katz, MD, is affiliated with the Department of OB/GYN, Division of Maternal-Fetal Medicine at the School of Medicine, University of North Carolina, Chapel Hill, NC 27599-7570.

Please send all request for reprints and correspondence to Vern L. Katz, MD, Department of OB/GYN, School of Medicine, CB# 7570, 214 MacNider Building, University of North Carolina, Chapel Hill, NC 27599-7570.

this new visualization. There is greater emphasis now on two patients, rather than on the mother alone.

The physician's increased reliance on ultrasound for clinical assessment, such as for gestational dating, assurance of fetal well-being, and placental localization, have redirected the focus of obstetrics. Additionally, prenatal diagnosis has become almost a specialty within itself as the development of high resolution ultrasound has enabled clinicians to count toes and measure intracerebral blood flow.

This essay will briefly review diagnostic ultrasound, its use in obstetrics, and its capabilities. The clinical applications in obstetrics will be outlined.

OBSTETRIC ULTRASOUND

Sound is a form of pressure that moves in a wave-like fashion, vibrating from one particle to another.[1,2] This property is important when sound is used for diagnostic purposes. For example, ultrasound energy is lost very rapidly when traversing air where particles are far apart. Thus, bowel gas in the abdomen inhibits imaging. Sound will travel at different speeds in different substances. By measuring the speed of travel one may infer what substances were penetrated. Diagnostic ultrasound relies on the ability of sound waves to bounce off structures and return to the transducer. This is the basic difference between diagnostic and therapeutic ultrasound. Diagnostic ultrasound is an analysis of the returning echoes.

The pulse of a sound wave is its frequency. High frequencies, greater than 20 cycles per second (or Hz) are too high for the human ear to hear, and thus have been defined as "ultrasound."[1,2] The range of diagnostic ultrasound is approximately 2.5 to 7 million cycles per second (MHz). The power or the intensity of diagnostic ultrasound is approximately .5 to 3 w/cm^2. The American Institute of Ultrasound in Medicine recommends 1 w/cm^2. Diagnostic ultrasound is from 20-100 times less powerful than therapeutic ultrasound, and exposure time is much less.[2] Because of the properties of sound waves, the higher the frequency the more detailed will be the echoes returning from nearby structures, and thus the greater the resolution of individual details. The higher the frequency, however, the less the distance the sound will penetrate.

The sound waves in a diagnostic ultrasound machine are produced by tiny crystals that are induced to vibrate by an electrical pulse. The quality of crystals to vibrate with an electric pulse is defined as "piezoelectric crystals." Originally such crystals were made of quartz but now are primarily synthetic. The sound waves from the crystals flow to the body and then bounce back off various structures. The returning sound waves are echoes. The returning sound stimulates the crystals to vibrate again and an electric pulse is given off, this time to a cable. The returning electric signals are integrated and analyzed by a large computer which comprises the bulk of the ultrasound machine. The actual sound pulse emitted from the crystals lasts 1 microsecond. Hundreds of pulses are given off each second. The time when the ultrasound crystal is not pulsing is the time when it is absorbing the returning signals.

Much of the terminology regarding ultrasound refers to the shapes of transducers and the way in which the message is being received. Transducers are arrays of piezoelectric crystals, and may be built in a multitude of shapes and sizes for whatever organ is to be viewed (Figure 1). One of the most common transducers is a curved transducer that has crystals which are rotated through a 60-90° arc. This transducer is called a *sector scanner*. The advantage of the small curved transducer is that it can visualize a wide arc from a small portal. This allows application of the transducer between ribs to look at the heart, or in a fontanelle of a newborn to look at the intracerebral ventricles. A *linear array* is an ultrasound transducer with crystals fixed in a line. In addition, transducers have different frequencies, most commonly 3.5 and 5 MHz. Higher frequency transducers, be they linear, sector, or curvilinear, are used for evaluation of pregnancies that are closer to the mother's skin, e.g., early pregnancies. This is because the higher frequency sound waves do not penetrate as deeply. The advantage of higher frequencies is better resolution.

Types of Diagnostic Ultrasound

A-mode ultrasound, the original non-pictorial ultrasound, is not used for obstetric purposes. B-mode ultrasound (brightness modulation) produces images compiled over a given area under the trans-

FIGURE 1. Transducers used for diagnostic ultrasound (Photo Courtesy of Corometrics Medical Systems, Inc., Wallingford, CT).

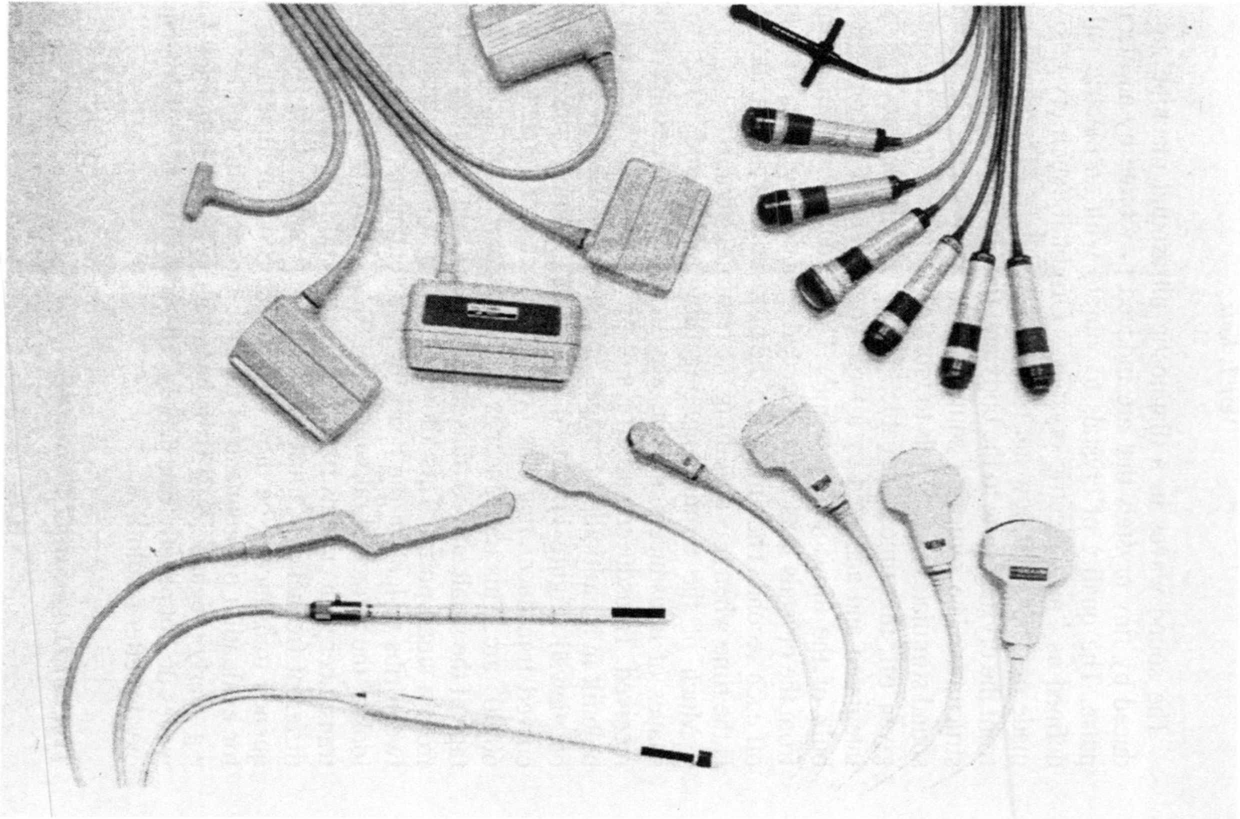

ducer. When multiple pulses and multiple echoes are sent and received, rather than one pulse with integration of one set of echoes, images will be seen to change shape as structures move under the transducer. This type of ultrasound is referred to as "real-time" B-mode. A single image is static B-mode, multiple images are real-time B-mode. As the computer integrates the echo signals, it reproduces the image on a TV monitor which is seen by the sonographer as well as the patient. The machine senses the different times for echoes to return, and uses that information to create a picture which represents the outline or shape of the internal area which is scanned. The details, for example, of a baby's face or hands are produced because the returning echoes bounce off the nose prior to bouncing off the eyes or lips. Again, when multiple shots of the hand are taken, we can follow the hand's motion over time. By studying the fetal movements we make assumptions about the physiologic aspects, health, and state of the organ being visualized or the fetus as a whole. For example, exposure to cigarette smoke produces an increase in fetal chest motion.

M-mode ultrasound is used to visualize movement within a single dimension over a period of time. For example, the valve motion of a heart can be seen to move up and down underneath the M-mode ultrasound transducer over a matter of time. If the movement is inappropriate, one might diagnose certain aspects of heart disease.

The ultrasound machine can measure not only the time when an ultrasound pulse echoes back, but also relative strength of the returning echo. From the strength of the returning echo, assumptions can be made about what structures the sound waves have passed through. For example, maximal return of an echo may represent a bone, whereas minimal return of an echo might represent a liquid, such as the amniotic fluid. The relative strengths of returning echoes is translated into different shades of gray on the TV monitor. This is known as *gray scale ultrasound*. Bones and cartilage are portrayed as very bright white, amniotic fluid is dark black, and the fat, liver, and cartilage are intermediate shades of gray. An air-filled bowel or air between the skin of the transducer may interfere with the picture and also be shown as dark black.

When an endovaginal ultrasound is performed, a thin transducer is placed in the vagina to visualize early pregnancies. The mother is usually in a dorsal lithotomy position. Endovaginal ultrasound is used for early pregnancy diagnosis because of the proximity of the transducer to small intrauterine structures (Figure 2). The disadvantage of endovaginal ultrasound is that it cannot visualize areas beyond the pelvis.[3] Thus, in advanced gestations when the fetus is intra-abdominal, endovaginal ultrasound is of little diagnostic help. However, endovaginal ultrasound may be helpful in visualizing premature dilatation of the cervix, or in localization of the placenta.

Doppler ultrasound is used primarily to evaluate blood flow either in the fetal cardiovascular system, or in the maternal uterine arteries. Doppler refers to the changes in frequency that occur when a wave bounces off a moving structure. This technique, which may be built into many current models of ultrasound machines, measures the change of sound wave frequencies as the sound waves reflect off of moving red blood cells within blood vessels. An abnormal Doppler examination indicates inappropriate velocities which may represent high resistance in the blood vessels. Certain disease states such as hypertension, or placental infarction, may lead to a back-up of blood, slow velocities, and abnormal Doppler examinations. Decreased diastolic flow in the fetal umbilical cord may represent placental pathology. Color Doppler may be superimposed on the regular Doppler to indicate areas of flow through the heart or umbilical cords, where none might be suspected. Color Doppler, therefore, interpolates color in the place of soundwaves. Interestingly, the frequency of the Doppler shift is in the range audible to humans and can be used to auscultate fetal heartbeats.

Continuous Doppler employs a steady emission from one piezoelectric crystal and a steady reception from another piezoelectric crystal. Continuous Doppler is inexpensive, but, unfortunately, will measure all signals from any moving structure beneath the Doppler transducer. Continuous Doppler is the technique used for fetal heart rate monitors for women in labor. Pulsed dopplers employ the real-time scanner to select an area of focus such as the fetal aorta and then measure flow within the specific area. Compared to continuous Dopplers, the hardware for the pulsed Doppler technique is more

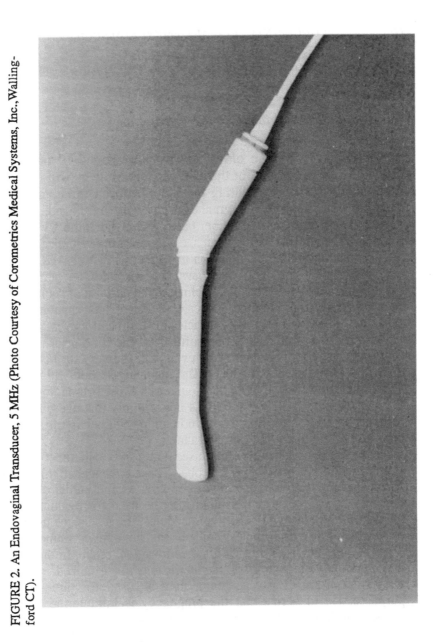

FIGURE 2. An Endovaginal Transducer, 5 MHz (Photo Courtesy of Corometrics Medical Systems, Inc., Wallingford CT).

expensive and requires extensive expertise to perform and interpret correctly.

Uses and Indications for Obstetric Ultrasound

A "routine" obstetric ultrasound usually takes 5-10 minutes, depending on the reason for the examination. Mothers will usually lie on their back or side during the examination. During an ultrasound examination the sonographer usually sits by the side of the patient. The patient, and often her partner, can watch the TV monitor and, unlike an X-ray, they can see what is being visualized.

A routine ultrasound examination usually costs between $200-250. Special examinations, also called *Level II ultrasounds*, are performed with high resolution expensive machines. The purpose of such Level II ultrasounds is to visualize intricate details of fetal anatomy and function, such as fetal cranial ventricles or fetal heart valves.

Obstetric ultrasound may be useful from the time prior to conception throughout pregnancy and even after delivery for help with delivery of the placenta (Table 1). The following section will present various indications of obstetric ultrasound as it is used chronologically from conception to delivery. This is not to imply that every patient receives an ultrasound for every indication. Neither is ultrasound used more frequently early in pregnancy.

Preconception. Ultrasound is used extensively in the field of infertility via the endovaginal probe. The advantage of this high frequency probe is its closeness to the ovaries and uterus offering high resolution image. Ultrasound may be used for evaluation of ovarian follicles during infertility procedures. It may also be used for harvesting of in-vitro follicles. Follicles that are a few millimeters in diameter may be visualized with the endovaginal probe. In the same way, very early pregnancies in the uterus may be visualized.

First Trimester. Early scanning may be used for three major purposes: (1) to verify that the pregnancy is intrauterine, (2) to assess viability, and (3) to date the pregnancy. Obstetricians often use ultrasound early in pregnancy to verify viability and assure that the pregnancy is intrauterine rather than ectopic. Pregnancies may be verified by the appearance of a gestational sac as early as 2 weeks after conception.[3] This is at the time of the missed period.

TABLE 1. Uses of Obsetetric Ultrasound

Preconception:	Infertility-Assisted Reproductive Techniques
First Trimester:	Verification of Intrauterine Pregnancy
	Viability Assessment
	Dating
	Structure Evaluation
	Guiding Diagnostic Procedures
Second Trimester:	Dating
	Growth Evaluation
	Anatomic Evaluation
	Guiding Diagnostic Procedures
	Placental Localization
Third Trimester:	Growth Evaluation
	Biophysical Assessment
	Anatomic Evaluation
	Guiding Diagnostic and Therapeutic Procedures
Post-Delivery:	Delivery of Placenta

The fetal yolk sac is apparent by 21 days after conception, and the first fetal cardiac motion is usually visible a few days later. The "fetal pole" has been seen as early as 5 1/2 weeks after the last menstrual period.[3]

When a patient presents with spotting, early first trimester ultrasound is useful to attempt visualization of a fetal heart beat. Approximately 40% of women will spot early in pregnancy. Twenty percent of all women, about half the women who spot, will proceed to miscarry. If a fetal heartbeat is seen, the chances for a continuing pregnancy are increased dramatically. If a heartbeat is seen at 6-9 weeks, only about 5-10% of women who spot will miscarry. If a heartbeat is seen at 9-12 weeks, only about 2% will go on to miscarry.

"Dating" of a pregnancy is a confusing issue. Gestational age usually refers to time from the last period. Fetal age is dated from conception. It is customary for obstetricians to date pregnancies by gestational age–conception plus two weeks after the last menstrual period. The "dating" of a pregnancy is accurate plus or minus less than one week during the first trimester. The term "dating" means a verification of gestational age.[1,3] The technique of dating a pregnancy assumes that the average fetus will have a specific size at any particular time during pregnancy. Early pregnancy dating is the most accurate because as pregnancy continues the range of average size expands greatly. For example, the 8-month-old fetus may be small or large, but still be 8 months in gestational age. The technique for early dating is measurement of the longest crown to rump length. Early ultrasound dating is valuable because as pregnancy continues, obstetricians need to know if the fetus is growing correctly. In addition, when pregnancies go beyond their due date, obstetricians need to know at what point to intervene. Some patients may have menstrual dates that indicate that they are 42-43 weeks, but may have ovulated late, or have irregular menstrual cycles and thus may not even be at their true due date.

A less common, but fourth purpose of obstetric ultrasound in the first trimester is fetal evaluation, occasionally used at 10-12 weeks. Patients who are at high risk for carrying a fetus with structural anomalies, such as mothers with a previous child with a neural tube defect, may have an early ultrasound to view fetal anatomy. Early anatomical assessment has a reasonable specificity, however, the sensitivity is limited. Early anatomical verification by ultrasound is limited in the sense that if an anomaly is visualized, such as an absent limb, as in caudal regression syndrome of diabetics, or cystic hygroma in Turner Syndrome, it is quite obvious. Anatomic lesions usually are more subtle, however, and can be better visualized later in the second trimester from 16-24 weeks.

Late in the first trimester ultrasound has been used to guide diagnostic procedures. From 9-11 weeks some patients elect to undergo a biopsy of the chorion, a procedure known as chorionic villi sampling (CVS). The purpose of CVS is to obtain cells of fetal origin for genetic and chromosomal analysis. The sonographer can view the pregnancy using an abdominal transducer while the physician guides the 16-gauge plastic catheter transcervically. Transabdominal CVS under direct ultrasound guidance is also available.

Second and Third Trimester. Ultrasounds are used in the second trimester primarily for gestational age assessment and fetal anatomic evaluation. During the period from 13-26 weeks the biparietal diameter (BPD) of the fetal head and fetal femur correlate within 10-14 days with the true gestational age. The second most common use of ultrasound at this time is fetal anatomic assessment. The anatomy of the fetus is best visualized in this trimester because the fetus is not too large and the amniotic fluid provides a window of contrast. Table 2 lists organ systems which are usually assessed by anatomic evaluation during this period. Of particular importance is the evaluation of the central nervous system and neural tube (Figure 3). Neural tube defects are one of the most common congenital defects and are screened for by alpha fetoprotein (AFP) levels. Spina bifida is manifested not only by distortion of the spinal cord, but also by notching of the fetal parietal bones, Arnold-Chiari malformation, and mild hydrocephalus (Figure 4). The fetal heart, stomach, kidneys, bladder, limbs, and face are also routinely visualized in the second trimester anatomic survey (Figures 5-7).

During the second trimester ultrasound may also be used for direct visualization and needle guidance of diagnostic procedures. Amniotic fluid may be aspirated for growth of cells in chromosomal, as well as genetic analysis. Down syndrome and other aneuploidies associated with increased maternal age are common indications for amniocentesis. Other reasons include evaluation of amniotic fluid for AFP to rule out neural tube defects, and evaluation for inherited genetic diseases such as cystic fibrosis or muscular dystrophy. Direct sampling of fetal blood cells for evaluation for both genetic and fetal chemistry and immunoglobulins may be accomplished by puncture of the fetal umbilical cord. Percutaneous umbilical blood sampling (PUBS) or cordocentesis has a risk of fetal loss of approximately one percent.

TABLE 2.   **Organ Systems and Exemplary Anomalies Commonly Visualized by Ultrasound**

<u>CENTRAL NERVOUS SYSTEM</u>

Neural Tube Defects
Hydrocephalus
Microcephaly

<u>HEART/CHEST</u>

Hypoplastic Left Heart
Diaphragmatic Hernia
Other Congenital Cardiac Defects

<u>ABDOMEN</u>

Omphalocoele
Hydronephrosis
Duodenal Atresia
Fetal Ovarian Follicles

<u>EXTREMITIES</u>

Intrauterine Growth Retardation
Dwarfism

<u>SKIN</u>

Hydrops
Cystic Hygroma

In the late second and third trimester, ultrasound has been used to guide placement of shunts to relieve fetal hydrocephalus or fetal hydronephrosis and megacystis. The purpose of this procedure is to relieve back pressure and let fluid drain into the amniotic cavity in order to release the pressure and allow for better development of brain or the kidneys, respectively. These procedures are rare and have been shown not to fulfill the promise they once were thought to possess.

Ultrasound is also used in the second and third trimesters for

FIGURE 3. Sonogram of a 16-week fetus with spina bifida. This is a longitudinal view of the spine. The arrow points to the widening in the lumbosacral spine.

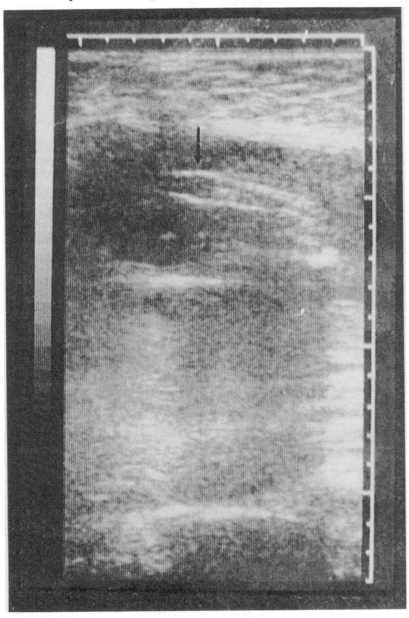

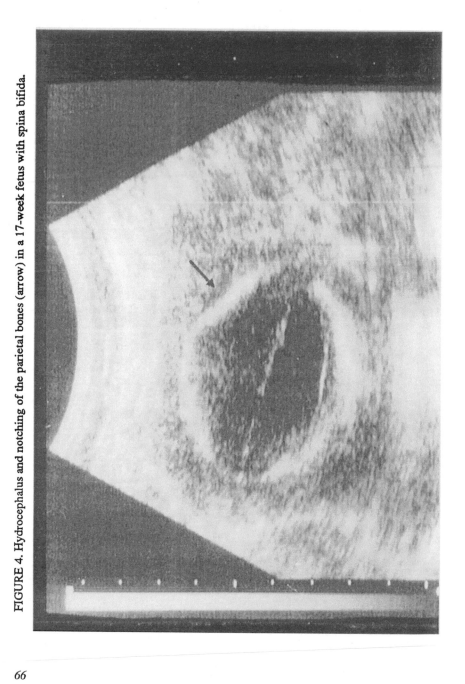

FIGURE 4. Hydrocephalus and notching of the parietal bones (arrow) in a 17-week fetus with spina bifida.

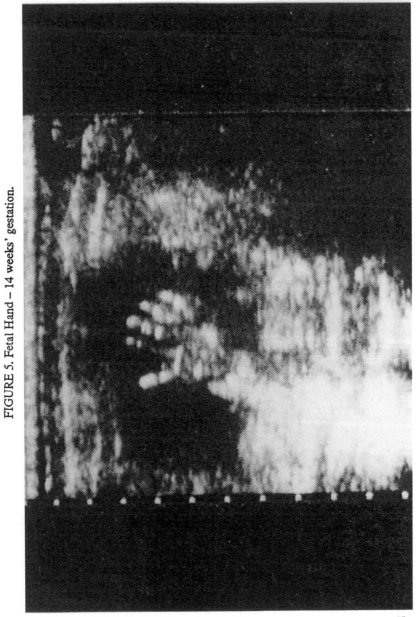

FIGURE 5. Fetal Hand – 14 weeks' gestation.

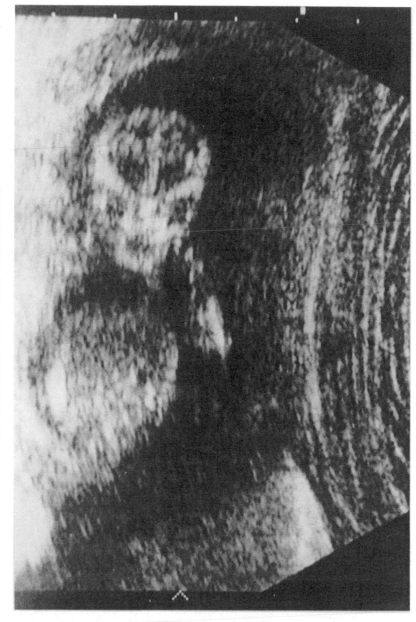

FIGURE 6. Frontal view of a 13-week fetal head.

FIGURE 7. Sonogram of transverse section of the fetal abdomen, 15 weeks gestation. Arrow points to the umbilical cord insertion. The twirling nature of the umbilical vessels can be appreciated in this view of a long segment of umbilical cord.

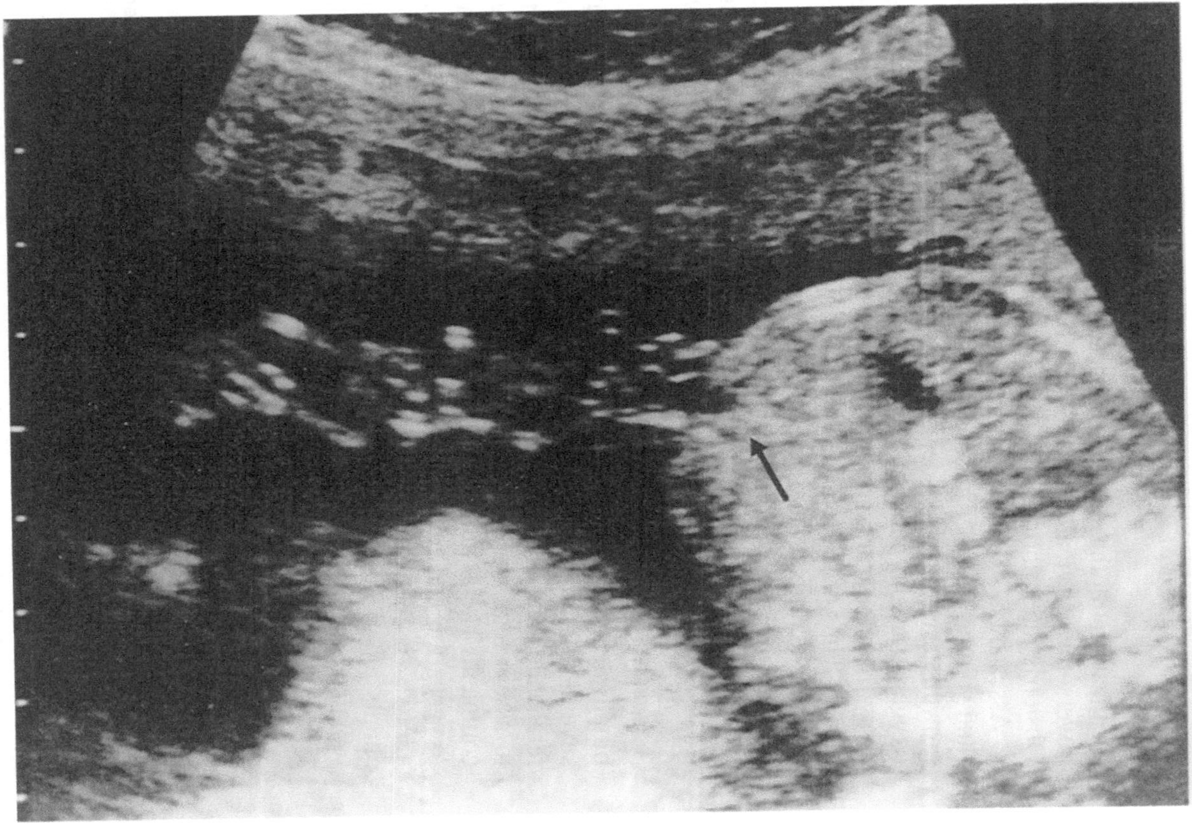

localization of the placenta. Placenta previa, where the placenta covers the cervical os, can lead to significant vaginal bleeding. Obstetric intervention is indicated when a placenta previa is found.

Assessment of growth of the fetus and quantification of amniotic fluid volume are other reasons for late pregnancy ultrasounds. Interval growth scans may help detect inadequacies in fetal nutrition. When oxygenation and nutrition are decreased, the fetus will shunt blood away from the trunk and limbs to the fetal brain, heart, and adrenal glands. Thus, if the fetal head is growing appropriately, but the fetal limbs or abdomen have grown poorly within a two-week span, the obstetrician may become suspicious of fetal growth retardation. Fetal growth retardation can occur for many different reasons, such as maternal hypertension, maternal vascular disease, or placental disease.

In the late second and third trimester, ultrasound is used for biophysical assessment. Biophysical assessment is an evaluation of several fetal characteristics which correlate with oxygenation and fetal state. The biophysical profile is the most commonly used tool to assess fetal well-being (Table 3) and takes up to 30 minutes to complete. The assumption behind biophysical assessment is that as oxygenation and nutrition decrease, the fetus' movements will be altered. As fetal oxygenation and nutrition decrease and the fetus shunts blood away from the fetal kidneys, amniotic fluid volume will decrease. As oxygenation continues to fall, fetal movement will

TABLE 3.   The Biophysical Profile

Score	Criteria
2	'Reactive' non-stress test: continuous ultrasound recording of the fetal heart rate, with heart rate accelerations during fetal movement.
2	Two episodes of fetal movement.
2	A 2 cm x 2 cm pocket of amniotic fluid.
2	Two episodes of fetal breathing motion.
2	Tone: movement of a fetal limb from flexion to extension with a return to flexion.

decline, and the fetal posture will change from generalized flexion to generalized extension. Fetal movements will also decrease with decreasing oxygenation.

Notation of a normal fetal heart rate of 120-160 BPM is insufficient alone to verify fetal health. It is the pattern of fetal heart rate that is of interest for the physician. With fetal movement or fetal stimulation, the fetal heart rate should accelerate. Occasionally, an artificial larynx will be used for acoustic stimulation of the fetus. It should produce a fetal heart rate acceleration and not produce a fetal heart rate deceleration. Analysis of fetal movement is of clinical as well as research interest. Fetal movement is often evaluated clinically to note the change from flexion to extension of limbs and fingers. This is valuable in diagnosing muscular diseases and certain chromosomal abnormalities.

OTHER CONCERNS
OF DIAGNOSTIC ULTRASOUND

Safety

The safety of ultrasound is discussed extensively later in this issue. Briefly, the potential biologic risks from ultrasound are related to the heating of tissue from the intensity, or power, of the sound waves, as well as the local disruption of tissue due to induced vibration, an effect known as *cavitation*.[4,5] In evaluating the safety of ultrasound we look at both the immediate effects or the long-term more subtle effects. In evaluating both short- and long-term effects, the amount of fetal exposure in a typical examination should be quantified.

Diagnostic ultrasound uses the pulsed technique as discussed above. The transducer is emitting sound waves only for a small fraction of the time it is turned on. The rest of the time it is receiving echoes. Thus, the true exposure is only a fraction of the total examination time. Andrews et al. evaluated the time of ultrasound exposure in a routine ultrasound examination. The mean time for a Level I ultrasound was 6 minutes and 46 seconds.[4] This calculated to a true maternal ultrasound exposure of 131 milliseconds. The fetus, depending on the gestational age, receives a fraction of this exposure. Most experiments using ultrasound have exposed animals to much greater amounts of ultrasound for much longer periods of time, such as daily exams for several weeks.[6,7] Results from clinical experiments on the short-term effects of ultrasound are, therefore, difficult to translate into the human experience. Two helpful studies evaluating long-term effects on humans have shown no difference in children exposed to in-utero ultrasound. One study examined sibling pairs for height, weight, and head circumference at 6 years of age.[8] This study found no difference in these factors. Investigators from Norway assessed children at 8-9 years of age whose mothers had participated in a study of routine ultrasound. Intelligence, performance at school, and reading and spelling skills were evaluated. There was no difference between the group exposed to antenatal ultrasound and controls.[9] Given the three decades of ultrasound use in modern obstetrics, no apparent deleterious effects have been seen in humans.

Psychological Effects

Several authors have commented on the profound effect of ultrasound on maternal attitudes.[10-15] Sonographers who perform obstetric ultrasound examinations frequently comment on the intense emotion of parents when viewing their baby. This profound and intense emotion not only carries over into the caregivers' attitude towards the pregnancy, but also is shared, in part, by sonographers in the way that they relate to the baby. It is not uncommon to watch sonographers initially start an examination by using the pronoun *it*, and convert to *he* or *she* when describing the fetus.

One of the most important aspects of the examination is communication between the person performing the ultrasound and the patient.[16] Heightened awareness on the part of the parents may easily lead to over-interpretation. A raised eyebrow and a worried sigh by the sonographer may create panic.[10,17-19] In another study, the most important and detrimental factor of obstetric ultrasound was found to be the failure of the ultrasound operator to communicate enough information to the parents.[13] In one study of women undergoing ultrasound with and without feedback from the sonographer, women with feedback had decreased anxiety, fewer obstetric complications, and infants with improved Brazelton neonatal assessments compared to women without feedback.[11] In contrast, Heidrich and Cranley did not find increased maternal attachment after routine ultrasound examination.[12]

Cost Effectiveness

The question of the cost effectiveness and value of routine ultrasound has been studied in several countries. The question is not ultrasound vs. no ultrasound, but routine ultrasound vs. a selective ultrasound for obstetric indications. In the studies of selective ultrasound vs. routine ultrasound, approximately 24-50 percent of pregnancies will end up having an ultrasound. It is difficult to estimate what percentage of women undergo ultrasounds currently in the United States. My estimation would put it between 70-80 percent of pregnancies. In the Helsinki ultrasound study, women with routine vs. selective ultrasound had an increased diagnosis of twins, a decreased overall perinatal mortality, and fewer visits to the clinic for other problems.[20] This last finding may be related to a greater sense of maternal well-being after the scan. Waldenstrom et al. from Stockholm noted fewer labor inductions, a decreased frequency of low birth weight infants, and an increased diagnosis of twins in the group with routine ultrasound.[21] In a study from Norway, Eik-Nes et al. found similar results.[22] Two additional studies from Sweden found similar improved outcomes and a general cost-benefit analysis in favor of routine ultrasound.[23,24] In studies from both Tucson, Arizona, and London, however, no improvement in neonatal outcome was noted with routine vs. selective ultrasound.[25-27] In current practice in most sections of the United States, ultrasound is not routine.

FUTURE DEVELOPMENT

The future development of ultrasound lies in two areas. The first is three-dimensional ultrasound. Several centers are working to produce a three-dimensional image (compared to the current two-dimensional image).[28] Such a three-dimensional image would significantly aid guidance of diagnostic procedures and enhance viewing for anatomic diagnoses. The effect of seeing the entire baby rather than just a slice or part of the fetus may have an impact on the parents.

Another important area of ultrasound development is the analysis of movement for assessment of fetal health and the developing nervous system. This monograph contains several reports regarding work in this area. More work needs to be done at all gestational ages regarding fetal movement and its relationship to the continuum of fetal health. No health provider would evaluate a patient by merely listening to the heartbeat. A patient's health is much better assessed by direct visualization of the person's activity and interaction with the environment. Additionally, the evaluation of fetal movement in substance abusers, in families at risk for having infants with neuromuscular disease, and in fetuses with structural abnormalities, is an area of much needed research.

REFERENCES

1. Seeds JW, Cefalo RC. *Practical Obstetrical Ultrasound*. Rockville, MD: Aspen Publications; 1986.

2. Ziskin MC. Basic physics of ultrasound. In: Fleischer AC, Romero R, Manning FA, Jeanty P, James AE, eds. *Ultrasonography in Obstetrics and Gynecology* 4th Edition. Norwalk, CT: Appleton and Lange; 1991, pp 1-14.

3. Goldstein SR. *Endovaginal Ultrasound* 2nd Edition. New York: Wiley-Liss; 1991.

4. Andrews M, Webster M, Fleming JEE, McNay MB. Ultrasound exposure time in routine obstetric scanning. *Br J Obstet Gynecol*. 1987; 94:843-846.

5. Meire HB. The safety of diagnostic ultrasound. *Br J Obstet Gynecol*. 1987; 94:1121-1122.

6. Ellisman MH, Palmer DE, Andre MP. Diagnostic levels of ultrasound may disrupt myelination. *Experimental Neurol*. 1987; 98:78-92.

7. Tarantal AF, Hendrickx. Evaluation of the bioeffects of prenatal ultrasound exposure in the cynomolgus maccaque (macaca fascicularis): II. Growth and behavior during the first year. *Teratology*. 1989; 39:149-162.

8. Lyons EA, Dyke C, Toms M, Cheang M. In utero exposure to diagnostic ultrasound: a 6-year follow-up. *Radiol*. 1988; 166:687-690.

9. Salvesen KA, Bakketeig LS, Eik-Nes SH, Undheim JO, Okland O. Routine ultrasonography in utero and school performance at age 8-9 years. *Lancet* 1992; 339:85-89.

10. Sparling JW, Seeds JW, Farran DC. The relationship of obstetric ultrasound to parent and infant behavior. *Obstet Gynecol.* 1988; 72:902-907.

11. Field T, Sandberg D, Quetel TA, Garcia R, Rosario M. Effects of ultrasound feedback on pregnancy anxiety, fetal activity, and neonatal outcome. *Obstet Gynecol.* 1985; 66:525-528.

12. Heidrich SM, Cranley MS. Effect of fetal movement, ultrasound scans, and amniocentesis on maternal-fetal attachment. *Nurs Res.* 1989; 38:81-4.

13. Hyde B. An interview study of pregnant women's attitudes to ultrasound scanning. *Soc Sci Med.* 1986; 22:587-592.

14. Tsoi MM, Hunter M, Pearce M, Chudleigh P, Campbell S. Ultrasound scanning in women with raised serum alpha fetoprotein: short term psychological effect. *J Psychosom Res.* 1987; 31:35-39.

15. Warsof SL, Pearce JM, Campbell S. The present place of routine ultrasound screening. *Clin Obstet Gynecol.* 1983; 10:445-457.

16. Garcia J, Corry M, MacDonald D, Elbourne D, Grant A. Mothers' views of continuous electronic fetal heart monitoring and intermittent auscultation in a randomized controlled trial. *Birth.* 1985; 12:79-86.

17. Griffiths DM, Gough MH. Dilemmas after ultrasonic diagnosis of fetal abnormality. *Lancet i.* 1985; 623-624.

18. Furness ME. Reporting obstetric ultrasound. *Lancet i.* 1987; 675-676.

19. Lind T. Obstetric Ultrasound: getting good vibrations. *Br Med J.* 1986; 293:576-577.

20. Saari-Kemppainen A, Karjalainen O, Ylostalo P, Heinonen OP. Ultrasound screening and perinatal mortality: controlled trial of systematic one-stage screening in pregnancy. *Lancet.* 1990; 336:387-391.

21. Waldenstrom U, Axelsson O, Nilsson S, Eklund G, Fall O, Lindeberg S, Sjodin Y. Effects of routine one-stage ultrasound screening in pregnancy: a randomized controlled trial. *Lancet.* 1988; 585-588.

22. Eik-Nes ST, Okland O, Aure JC. Ultrasound screening in pregnancy: A randomized controlled trial. *Lancet.* 1984; 1347.

23. Persson PH, Kullander S. Long-term experience of general ultrasound screening in pregnancy. *Am J Obstet Gynecol.* 1983; 146:942-947.

24. Belfrage P, Fernstrom I, Hallenberg G. Routine or selective ultrasound examinations in early pregnancy. *Obstet Gynecol.* 1987; 69:747.

25. Thacker SB. Quality of controlled clinical trials. The case of imaging ultrasound in obstetrics: a review. *Br J Obstet Gynecol.* 1985; 92:437-444.

26. Bennett MJ, Little G, Dewhurst SJ, Chamberlain G. Predictive value of ultrasound measurement in early pregnancy: a randomized controlled trial. *Br J Obstet Gynecol.* 1982; 89:338-341.

27. Ewigman B, LeFevere M, Hesser J. A randomized trial of routine prenatal ultrasound. *Obstet Gynecol.* 1990; 76:189.

28. Ohbuchi R, Fuchs H. Incremental 3D ultrasound imaging from a 2D scanner. To appear in Proceedings of the "First Conference on Visualization in Biomedical Computing." May 22-25, 1990, Atlanta, GA.

Ultrasound Safety:
A Descriptive Study
of the Potential Effects of Early Imaging

LB Tucker
WR Gentry
EA Thomas
JW Sparling

SUMMARY. Animal and human research is reviewed to clarify the current understanding of the safety of obstetric ultrasound. As an obligation to subjects who are volunteering to participate in research on fetal movement, a follow-up study of seven subjects who received serial ultrasound in utero is described. Results suggest that there is no effect of diagnostic ultrasound imaging on the motor development of toddlers who received ultrasound in utero.

THE PROBLEM

Obstetric ultrasound imaging is a routine procedure. Its use among women with live births has increased in the United States

LB Tucker, WR Gentry, and EA Thomas are affiliated with clinical sites in Winston-Salem, NC, Nashville, TN, and Roanoke, VA. JW Sparling, PhD, PT, OT, is Assistant Professor in the Division of Physical Therapy at the University of North Carolina at Chapel Hill. She is Project Director for the Maternal and Child Health Postgraduate Training Grant.

Funded in part by a Department of Health and Human Services, Maternal and Child Health Training Grant 149, an Innovative Research Award from Frank Porter Graham Research Center, and a Department of Medical Allied Health Professions Grant, University of North Carolina at Chapel Hill.

Paper presented in partial fulfillment for a Bachelor of Science degree in Physical Therapy at the University of North Carolina at Chapel Hill.

from 33.5 percent in 1980 to 78.8 percent in 1987.[1] Definitive statements about the safety of this diagnostic procedure, however, are lacking. At least three factors are involved in determining the safety of ultrasound with human subjects: little systematic research exists on humans exposed to ultrasound;[2] equipment and procedures related to ultrasound use have not been adequately standardized;[3] and ethical concerns related to the sharing of ultrasound information are extensive.[4]

Data on the safe use of ultrasound have not been readily available. Over twenty years after its commercial introduction, the measurement, applications and biological effects of ultrasound were published by the Center for Devices and Radiological Health.[5] Similar delay characterized the development and use of X-ray technology. This fact has promoted a demand for research on the safety of ultrasound, a demand supported by the American College of Obstetricians and Gynecologists.[6]

In addition to the lack of research, the use of ultrasound imaging equipment has not been sufficiently scrutinized. Until recently, imaging equipment and protocols for its use were not standardized because the benefit of diagnosis was thought to be greater than any potential for harm.[7] Diagnosing multiple fetuses or fetal demise, confirming gestational age and placental location, and determining a baseline for later fetal growth add dramatically to the effectiveness of prenatal and perinatal care. An additional benefit is the early diagnosis of abnormalities and the resultant savings in health care costs.[7,8] That ultrasound is beneficial is not in doubt. The question of its safety arises with the knowledge that the intensity of any "dose" can be increased by modifying the focus, amplitude or duration of application.[3] According to the American Institute of Ultrasound in Medicine, the accepted intensity should be no greater than 100 mW/cm^2.[9] Additional concern exists with the advent of newer imaging approaches,[10] such as transvaginal scanning and chorionic villus sampling. These procedures require earlier use of ultrasound during the period of organogenesis and nervous system development and suggest a potential for harm.

A number of ethical issues arise in the use of ultrasound in obstetrics. Chervenak and McCullough[4] describe four major concerns, including the competence of examiners, routine use of ultrasound, disclosure of results, and confidentiality. Competent examiners diagnose and sensitively explain for the concerned mother the fetal conditions being observed and the safety of the procedure. A discussion of safety could include the different types of high frequency sound beyond the human audible range of 20,000 Hertz (Hz) or cycles per second. Diagnostic ultrasound frequencies extend over a small part of that range from 2.5 to 7.0 million Hertz, i.e., 2.5-5.0 MHz. In contrast, therapeutic ultrasound uses higher frequencies for the purpose of heating and destroying tissue. The wide and sometimes indiscriminate use of ultrasound is a concern of the competent ultrasonographer and exists not only in the United States but has been documented internationally, with at least 82 percent of French women having a one to three stage ultrasound scan during pregnancy.[2] Finally, the ultrasonographer should be committed to maintaining the confidentiality of patient information.

The purpose of this paper is to review research that describes the safety controversy and to present a long-term follow-up of seven subjects who received serial obstetric ultrasound imagings early in pregnancy. The review includes animal as well as human research. The follow-up study uses motor development as the outcome variable and as a marker of the status of the central nervous system.[11]

REVIEW OF LITERATURE

Ultrasound uses high frequency sound waves to form an image of the fetus (See Katz's article in this issue for further information). Because no ionizing radiation is involved, it has been considered a safe procedure. The most comprehensive reviews of obstetric ultrasound[6,12,13] support this determination and conclude that under controlled applications, the woman and her fetus do not experience harmful effects. Animal research, however, has resulted in some disturbing findings that have perpetuated the dialogue on ultrasound safety.

Two biologic mechanisms for potentially harmful effects are heating and cavitation. Although the heating of amniotic fluid and fetal tissues has been shown to be minimal,[14] potential heating can be better controlled by using low spatial and temporal intensities.

When low intensities are used, heating is diminished, if not eliminated, as a causative factor and cavitation remains the major potential source of danger. Cavitation refers to the "interactions of a sound field with microscopic gas bodies in the exposed medium."[15,p598] Little is known about cavitation in mammals, but lower level organisms exposed to low temporal, average intensity ultrasound have shown some deleterious effects on their infant neurologic, immunologic, hematologic, developmental and genetic systems.[9] These potential consequences of ultrasound exposure warrant an overview of animal and human research related to ultrasound safety.

Animal Research

Fruit flies (Drosophilia). The response of Drosophilia to ultrasound has been studied in all four stages of development: eggs, larvae, pupae and adult flies. Child, Carstensen and Lam[16] exposed larvae to 2.5 minutes of pulsed-echo diagnostic ultrasound that resulted in a sharp threshold for killing larvae between temporal maximum intensities of 10-20 W/cm^2. Fruit fly eggs showed a slightly higher threshold response than flies in later stages of development. The results are some of the strongest available evidence that this type of exposure can cause adverse biological effects. The intensities of the exposure, however, were markedly higher than the maximum intensities of 100 mW/cm^2 used with humans.

Rodents. More recently, Ellisman, Palmer, and Andre[17] investigated the effects of diagnostic ultrasound on the myelination of neonatal rats. The rat pup age of 3-5 days was studied because myelination in the neonatal rat is similar to that of the human fetus of 4-5 months, a time during which ultrasound is commonly used in humans. Litters of 8-10 rat pups were randomly divided into exposed and non-exposed groups. The experimental rats were bound and exposed to ultrasound for 30 minutes, while the non-exposed rats were simply bound. Thirty hours after exposure, the dorsal nerve roots were examined by electron microscopy and revealed disruption of the nodes of Ranvier in the exposed group. The intensities used in this study were similar to those employed in human imaging. Whether these effects were transient is not known.

Low birth weight was identified as one of the first significant biological effects of diagnostic ultrasound. O'Brien[18] reported a significant dose-dependent effect of fetal weight reduction in mice when exposed to 0.5-5.5 W/cm^2 (10-300 secs), but using another strain of mice, he was unable to replicate these results. In a more recent study, no long-term negative effect of ultrasound on birth weight was reported.[19]

In an earlier investigation,[20] a higher temporal peak intensity of 1900 W/cm^2 compared to 600 W/cm^2 resulted in more fetal abnormalities, resorption and decreased litter size. Inconsistencies in study results may well be due to the lack of consistency in study design and implementation, such as differences in intensities.

Additional studies of ultrasound effects using rodents include the immune system and depression of phagocytosis,[21] cell motility of rat fibroblasts exposed in vitro,[22] the development of lymphocytes,[23] and premature death and malformations.[24] Studies using conditions similar to human imaging show no negative effects of obstetric ultrasound.

Primates. Perhaps the most interesting nonhuman study regarding biological effects of ultrasound was conducted with the Cynomolgus Macque.[25] In this study, researchers used a commercial real-time scanner to expose non-human primates to ultrasound at 12 mW/cm^2, for 10 minutes weekly, from gestational age 21 to 150 days. A total of 13 exposed and 10 non-exposed animals completed all the phases of testing. Several other subjects were eliminated from study due to premature delivery and sickness. The exposed animals showed lower birth weight and white blood cell counts, shorter crown-rump lengths, and higher Apgar muscle tone and color scores. The reduction in body weight and the hematologic changes were still significant at three months, but no long-term effect at 12 months was found.

This study also included a series of behavioral evaluations based on a neurobehavioral test battery. Results showed increased muscle tone in exposed monkeys at one, two and four days. In infancy,[26] the exposed animals displayed more quiet-type activities than the controls. Although no group differences were noted in discrimination learning, group differences in performances of motor and cognitive tasks were observed. These differences may have been attributable, however, to agitation and difficulty in adjusting to the test environment.

The authors conclude that the effects of real-time ultrasound are probably transitory with less than maximum acoustic power output of 12 mW/cm^2 and duration of 20 minutes. The frequency of exposures in this study (three times each week) was notably greater than in normative human obstetric imaging, however, making comparisons to humans inappropriate.

Human Research

Although useful investigations can be conducted with small animals as experimental models, clinical techniques must ultimately be evaluated with human subjects.[27, 28] Potential clinical signs of prenatal use of ultrasound with humans include decreased weight and height, structural anomalies, delayed neurologic development, neoplasms, dyslexia, hearing disorders, and behavioral deviations.

Weight and height. Numerous studies on weight and height have been conducted since the early use of obstetric ultrasound. Two long-term investigations suggest no effect of imaging on birth weight. In a review of cases from 1975-1983,[29] an analysis was conducted of 149 sibling pairs of the same sex, one of whom had been exposed to diagnostic ultrasound in utero. The control group consisted of the unexposed siblings. Average duration of exposure was estimated at 20 minutes and the spatial peak, temporal average intensity ranged from .004-.028 W/cm^2. Results indicated no statistically significant differences in either weight or height between exposed and unexposed siblings from birth to six years of age.

Another long-term follow-up study, often referred to as the "Denver study,"[30] included a sample of 425 children exposed to diagnostic ultrasound and 381 matched control children who received no obstetric ultrasound. Through use of a ranking procedure conducted by obstetricians and pediatricians at birth and at 7 and 12 years of age, no difference was found between the control and experimental group on weight and height. These data are encouraging. Even with large population studies, however, it is difficult to detect "small increases in the rate of a commonly occurring event, . . . subtle effects such as minor chemical changes and minor behavioral changes, or long-term delayed effects."[28,p96]

Structural anomalies. No effect of ultrasound imaging has been reported on the prevalence of structural anomalies.[31, 32] The results of these early studies from the 1970's have been supported by research conducted in the 1980's.[29, 33] In one of these studies,[29] only 13% of the subjects were exposed to ultrasound during the period of organogenesis. Because organogenesis is complete prior to the most common use of ultrasound with amniocentesis at 14-16 weeks, structural deviations have not been associated with prenatal exposure to ultrasound. With ultrasound being used earlier in conjunction with chorionic villus sampling, further study on safety is still suggested.

Neurologic development. During this early period from 10-12 weeks of gestation, potential damage may occur to the migration of neurons and the development of the cerebral hemispheres. In a retrospective follow-up of 303 ultrasound-exposed children and 931 unexposed children,[32] and in the Denver study,[30] ultrasound was not associated with negative neurological developmental outcomes. In the Denver study, however, a 4.7 percent increase in the incidence of dyslexia was reported in the ultrasound group when compared to the control group.

Other potential effects. In the Denver study, no difference was found in the number of ear infections at ages 7-12 years, nor in the hearing of children because of ultrasound exposure. In addition, no consistent or significant evidence existed on measures of task orientation, dependency, distractibility, and intelligence.[30] Other investigations have shown no relationship between ultrasound and childhood cancer.[34,35]

Movement. Only three studies have specifically addressed the effect of ultrasound on fetal movement. David et al.[36] reported increased movement of the human fetus using Doppler ultrasound. Two later studies[37,38] were unable to document this effect. If movement were affected either directly or indirectly by ultrasound, the effect might be observed in the lack of variability and coordination of movement patterns, factors known to be associated with movement abnormalities.[39] To date this effect has not been observed.

Limitations of Previous Studies

In summary, no long-term negative effects have been shown with humans who have been exposed to judicious use of obstetric imaging.

Most of the early studies were designed inadequately, the procedures used were significantly different from actual diagnostic ultrasound imaging with humans, and information on exposure conditions was lacking.[40-42] In some studies, sample sizes were inadequate and follow-up was limited. The question of the harm/benefit ratio persists, however, because of the lack of design consistency among studies and the variability in equipment and its use. Because of the persisting commentaries and dictums related to ultrasound safety,[1-9] and the responsibility assumed in conducting ultrasound research, long-term follow-up of our subjects was considered an obligation.

METHOD

Subjects

Seven Caucasian children between the ages of 17 and 30 months (mean = 23 months) were evaluated in this follow-up study. The mothers of these toddlers had volunteered to participate in an earlier study of fetal movement[43] and received 30 minutes of diagnostic ultrasound every two weeks from 12-18 weeks of gestation. Of the original 10 subjects with toddlers appropriate for follow-up testing, two could not be located, and one was not interested in developmental follow-up in the home.

The mean age of the mothers at identification was 31.6 years, and for fathers was 33.7 years. The parents' grade level completed was over 18 years. All mothers worked outside of the home. Their jobs along with their spouses' occupations placed them in Hollingsheads' highest socioeconomic category. The mothers experienced a low-risk pregnancy, were non-smokers and drank only occasionally, if at all, during pregnancy.

Toddler subject data are shown in Table 1. There were three boys and four girls. Five out of the seven children were born prematurely at 34 to 37 weeks gestational age, with a mean birthweight of 2448 grams. The two full term infants were born at 40 weeks and had a mean birth weight of 3902 grams. At follow-up, the seven subjects were performing within normal limits according to maternal and pediatric report. Their educational placement at this time was a home- or center-based setting (Table 2).

Table 1. Birth Data of Seven Subjects Who Received
Serial Ultrasound Imaging at 12, 14, and 16 Weeks
of Gestation

Subject	Gender	Age at Birth (in weeks)	Weight at Birth (in grams)
1	F	37	2835
2	M	40	3402
3	M	35	2100
4	F	34	1928
5	M	37	3062
6	F	40	4400
7	F	36	2313
Mean		37	2863

Instrumentation

The Peabody Developmental Motor Scales (PDMS)[44] were used
to evaluate each toddler's motor performance. The PDMS, published in 1983, is a standardized, individually-administered test to
measure motor skill of children from birth to seven years of age.
The test is both norm-referenced and criterion-referenced and involves observation as well as handling of the child. The current
version of the PDMS has a Gross Motor and a Fine Motor Scale.
The Gross Motor Scale consists of 170 items divided into 17 age
levels and involves tasks that require precise movements related to
five skill categories: reflexes, balance, nonlocomotor, locomotor,
and receipt and propulsion of objects. The Fine Motor Scale has 112
items divided into 16 age levels and involves tasks that require
precise movements related to four skill categories: grasping, hand

Table 2.   Follow-up Data of Seven Subjects According to
Chronological Age, Gross and Fine Motor Age Equivalents at
Peabody Developmental Scale Testing and Subjects' Daily
Educational Setting

Subjects	Age at Testing (months)	GM Age Equiv. (months)	FM Age Equiv. (months)	Educational Setting
1	30	24	25	Home
2	23	26	23	Center
3	17	19	20	Home
4	28	22	28	Center
5	19	17	20	Center
6	17	18	17	Home
7	29	26	28	Center
Mean	23	22	23	

use, eye-hand coordination, and manual dexterity. Each of these
skill items are scored on a 3-point scale: "0"–the child can not or
will not attempt the behavior; "1"–the child's movement re-
sembles, but does not meet the criterion for the full test item; or
"2"–the child performs the item behavior to the criterion.

   The test was normed on 617 children of mixed ethnicity and
gender. Forty-two percent of these subjects were two years old or
less, providing a larger sample of children in this age category than
in the older categories, thus making it a particularly appropriate test
for our toddler sample. Test-retest reliability with 38 children was
.95 for the Gross Motor Scale and .80 for the Fine Motor Scale.
Interrater reliability with 36 children was .97 for Gross Motor and

.94 for Fine Motor. The PDMS was found to discriminate 104 developmentally delayed children from the normative values established for the scale, at all ages except 0-5 months.

The Parental Interview Questionnaire was developed by the investigators for the purpose of identifying demographic and ultrasound variables. These variables included toddler and parent ages, parental socioeconomic status, working history of the mother, complications of pregnancy, dates of ultrasound imagings, and learning and play environment of the child.

Procedure

Parental consent was initially obtained by a phone call from the principal investigator of the original study. All subjects contacted agreed to the follow-up assessment, although one subject did not appear to want a home visit and avoided study inclusion. The Parental Interview Questionnaire was completed by one researcher in the child's home after parental consent for participation was obtained. The PDMS was given by a second researcher. The interview and testing lasted approximately one and one-half hours. The same toys, as described in the Peabody Manual, were used in each home testing.

Analysis

The Friedman's non-parametric test[45] was applied to the raw data to determine any significant differences between chronological age and gross or fine motor age. Percentile ranks were obtained for each skill level and normalized T-scores were calculated for gross motor and fine motor areas according to the Peabody norms. The T-score represents the transformation of the raw score into a distribution with a mean of 50 and a standard deviation of 10, permitting comparison of subjects on overall gross and fine motor scale performance. For establishing statistical significance, a .05 alpha level was used that corresponds to a 1.65 standard deviation.[44,p125]

RESULTS

Results indicated no significant difference between the chronological age of the toddlers at the time of testing and the age-equivalent scores computed from the gross and fine motor sections of the PDMS (Table 2). The Chi square statistic was .93 (df = 2) with > 5.99 required to achieve significance. The mean Gross Motor age-equivalent score for the seven subjects was one month below the actual chronological age, while the mean Fine Motor score was the same as the actual mean age for the group.

Percentile ranks for gross and fine motor domains for the seven subjects are shown in Figure 1. Subjects 1 and 5 scored at the 23rd percentile or less; subject 4 was at the 25th percentile in the gross motor domain but in the 73rd percentile in the fine motor area. The discrepancy between gross motor and fine motor scores for all subjects is presented in Table 3 according to the normalized T-scores. Subject 4 showed the greatest discrepancy with a standard deviation of 1.3, still within our pre-established .05 level for the normal range. Subjects 1 and 5 scored the lowest in the gross motor domain with standard deviations of − 1.6 suggesting a borderline performance using the pre-established standard deviation of 1.65. All other scores were within the 1.65 cutoff for the normal range.

DISCUSSION

Results of this study indicate no significant difference in gross and fine motor skill scores between toddler's actual age and their age equivalency as determined by motor development test performance. Toddlers exposed to ultrasound in utero performed within a wide range of normal according to the normative data of the PDMS. The three toddlers with the lowest gross motor scores were all born prematurely. Of the two toddlers born at 37 weeks of gestation, one was female (subject 1) and one was male (subject 5); both had the lowest gross and fine motor scores. The other low gross motor score was for subject 4, a preterm female born at 34 weeks of gestation. Subjects 3 and 7, the remaining two premature infants, performed well within the normal ranges.

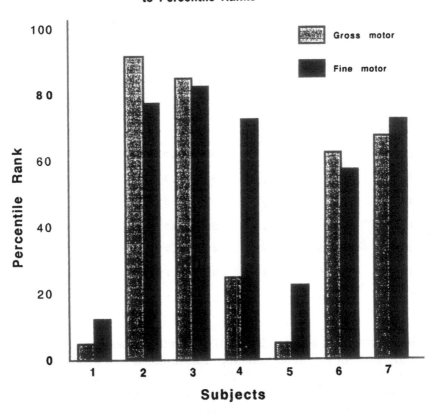

Figure 1 - Peabody Developmental Motor Scale Scores for Seven Subjects According to Percentile Ranks

The literature has suggested some long-term effects of prematurity that could explain the lower developmental scores. In a study of 97 high-risk preterm toddlers compared to 94 healthy full term toddlers, fine motor and adaptive skills were significantly delayed in 14 of 50 behaviors for the preterm children, who also attained over 80 percent of the developmental fine motor tasks later than the full term children.[46] Forslund and Bjerre have reported normal growth and development of preterms at four years of age, but described the preterm toddlers as physically smaller and performing less well

Table 3.   Peabody Developmental Motor Scale Gross Motor and
Fine Motor Normalized T-Scores and Standard Deviations for
Seven Subjects

	Normalized T-Scores		
Subjects	Gross Motor (SD)	Fine Motor (SD)	Differences
1	34 (−1.6)	38 (−1.2)	0.4
2	63 (1.3)	57 (0.7)	0.6
3	61 (1.1)	59 (0.9)	0.2
4	43 (−0.7)	56 (0.6)	1.3
5	34 (−1.6)	43 (−0.7)	0.9
6	53 (0.3)	52 (0.2)	0.1
7	55 (0.5)	56 (0.6)	0.1

than normal full term children on intellectual assessment.[47] In our study, low but within normal range fine motor scores were noted for subjects 1 and 5 who were born at 37 weeks of gestation. Neither the lowest fine or gross motor scores of our subjects were related to gender, although an increased frequency of neurological problems for males has been noted in the literature.[48]

Score differences for preterms have been related to social factors of the mother, such as her educational level.[49] This was not the case in our sample with all mothers in the highest educational categories. The effects of prematurity have been noted in characteristics of the child, such as more difficult temperaments. In one study,[50] 45 preterms of low medical risk were compared to 23 healthy full term infants. The preterms fussed and cried more, were harder to soothe when they cried than the full terms, and changed state more frequently. The authors suggested that these temperament characteristics could threaten the parent-child relationship and result in long-term performance differences between preterm and full term children.

Birth weight can be a confounding variable with prematurity. The mean weight at birth for the preterm infants in this study was 2448 grams, designating them as low-birth-weight newborn infants. Early investigations of low-birth-weight humans indicated no effect of ultrasound on birth weight.[31,32] Later studies with human subjects randomly assigned to two groups of ultrasound and no-ultrasound[33] also reported no effect on birth weight and height. Although differences may be too subtle to evaluate,[28] birth weight does not appear to be related to ultrasound exposure.

In our study, no findings were related to the placement of the child in day care or at home. The kind of learning opportunities that were available in these settings appeared to be very different, however, as did the interaction of the mother and child. For example, one child with decreased gross motor scores (subject 1) had less daily opportunity for gross motor experience than the other children. One parent experienced a divorce during the intervening months with some disorganization of routines noted by the examiner. No child injuries or hospitalizations occurred accounting for performance differences. Assessment of child or parent temperament, however, was not conducted.

Benefits of ultrasound imaging were reported by all parents who prospectively and retrospectively exuded pleasure with the experience. The ultrasound gave them an opportunity to become assured of their child's health and initiate interaction with their fetus.

Limitations of the study include the lack of a control group without exposure to ultrasound, that would have made blind testing with the Peabody a possibility. According to the impressive increase in the use of ultrasound in the last decade,[1,2] however, it is nearly impossible to obtain a control group that has not been exposed to ultrasound. The small number of subjects, in addition, is a major study limitation and precludes the generalization of these data.[40] Another potential influence on study results was the testing site. All subjects were tested in the natural environment of the child. A variety of distractions presented themselves during testing in the home and could have affected concentration on the test tasks. These distractions appeared normal to the child, however, and could have relaxed the toddler and supported a "best performance." Finally, it may be that either the PDMS may not be sensitive enough or motor development itself may not be a sufficient characteristic to determine the effect of diagnostic ultrasound.

FUTURE STUDY

This pilot study attempted to assess the long-term effects of serial ultrasound imaging in utero on the motor development of the young child. No definitive effects of imaging can be reported, although a wide normal variation occurred in the test scores. With the continued discussion of ultrasound safety, our investigators assumed an obligation to conduct a follow-up study.

Definitive results related to the safety of ultrasound imaging will continue to be difficult to obtain due to the enormous number of potential intervening variables that occur between imaging in utero and later performance. If future studies are to be conducted, they should include careful documentation of intervening variables and a serial follow-up from birth, to 3, 6, 9 and 12 months, and each year until the children attain school age. Some performance deficits do not show up until school structure and scheduling place additional performance demands on children. A variety of assessments including those aimed at detecting processing as well as motor skills, i.e., Miller Assessment for Preschoolers,[48] might provide more information on functional movement within a learning environment.

REFERENCES

1. Moore RM, Jeng LL, Kaczmarek RG, Placek PJ. Use of diagnostic imaging procedures and fetal monitoring devices n the care of pregnant women. *Public Health Reports.* 1990; 105(5):471-475.

2. Ringa V, Blondel B, Breart G. Ultrasound in obstetrics: do published evaluative studies justify its routine use? *Int J Epidem.* 1989;18(3):489-497.

3. Taylor KJW. A prudent approach to ultrasound imaging of the fetus and newborn. *Birth.* 1990;17(4):218-223.

4. Chervenak FA, McCullough LB. Ethics in obstetric ultrasound. *J Ultrasound Med.* 1989;8:493-497.

5. Stewart HF, Moore RM. Development of health risk evaluation data for diagnostic ultrasound: an historical perspective. *J Clin Ultrasound.* 1984; 12:493-500.

6. American College of Obstetricians and Gynecologists. *Ultrasound in pregnancy.* Technical Bulletin No.116. Chicago, IL: ACOG; 1988.

7. Wells PNT. The prudent use of diagnostic ultrasound. *Ultrasound Med Biol.* 1987;13(7):391-400.

8. Medical Research Council. Report on an ad hoc meeting to discuss the risks and benefits of obstetrical ultrasound. London: MRC; 1986.

9. American Institute of Ultrasound in Medicine. Bioeffects considerations for the safety of diagnostic ultrasound. *J Ultrasound Med.* 1988;7:S1-38.

10. Brambati B, Tului L, Simoni G, Travi M. Genetic diagnosis before the eighth gestational week. *Obstet Gynecol.* 1991;77(2):318-321.

11. Touwen BCL. Motility in the fetus and young infant: implications for neurological development. *Eur J Clin Nutr.* 1989;43:27-32.

12. Carstensen EL, Gates AH. The effects of pulsed ultrasound on the fetus. *J Ultrasound Med.* 1984;3:145-147.

13. Reese EA, Assimakopoulos E, Zheng X, Hagay Z, Hobbins JC. The safety of obstetric ultrasonography: concern for the fetus. *Obstet Gynecol.* 1990;76: 139-146.

14. Soothill PW, Nicolaides KH, Rodeck CH, Campbell S. Amniotic fluid and fetal tissues are not heated by obstetric ultrasound scanning. *Br J Obstet Gynecol.* 1987;94:675-677.

15. Carstensen EL. Acoustic cavitation and the safety of diagnostic ultrasound. *Ultrasound Med Biol.* 1987;13(10):597-606.

16. Child SZ, Carstensen EL, Lam SK. Effects of ultrasound on Drosophilia: III. Exposure of larvae to low-temporal-average-intensity, pulsed irradiation. *Ultrasound Med Biol.* 1981;7:167-173.

17. Ellisman MH, Palmer DE, Andre MP. Diagnostic levels of ultrasound may disrupt myelination. *Exp Neurol.* 1987;98(1):78-92.

18. O'Brien WD. Dose-dependent effect of ultrasound on fetal weight in mice. *J Ultrasound Med.* 1983;2:1-8.

19. Child SZ, Hoffman D, Strassner D, Carstensen EL, Gates AH, Cox C et al. A test of I^2T as a dose parameter for fetal weight reduction from exposure to ultrasound. *Ultrasound Med Biol.* 1989;15(1):39-44.

20. Fry FJ, Erdmann WA, Johnson LK, Baird AI. Ultrasonic toxicity study. *Ultrasound Med Biol.* 1978;3:351-366.

21. Anderson DW, Barrett JT. Ultrasound: a new immunosuppressant. *Clin Immunol Immunopathol.* 1979;14:18-29.

22. Liebeskind D, Padawar J, Wolley R, Bases R. Diagnostic ultrasound: time-lapse and transmission electron microscope studies of cells insonated in vitro. *Br J Cancer.* 1982;45 (Suppl.5):176-186.

23. Child SZ, Carstensen EL, Gates AH, Hall WJ. Testing for the teratogenicity of pulsed ultrasound in mice. *Ultrasound Med Biol.* 1988;14:493-498.

24. Desai BB, Sosolik RC, Ciaravino V, Teale JM. Effect of fetal exposure to ultrasound on the development of functional, antigen-specific B lymphocytes in fetal and neonatal balb/c mice. *Ultrasound Med Biol.* 1989;15(6):575-580.

25. Tarantal AF, Hendrickx SG. Evaluation of the bioeffects of prenatal ultrasound exposure in the cynomolgus macaque (Macaca fascicularis): I. Neonatal/infant observations. *Teratology.* 1989;39:137-147.

26. Tarantal AF, Hendrickx SG. Evaluation of the bioeffects of prenatal ultrasound exposure in the cynomolgus macaque (Macaca fascicularis): II. growth and behavior during the first year. *Teratology.* 1989;39:149-162.

27. Determining risk to subjects: exposure to ultrasound. *IRBA Review of Human Subjects Research.* 1987;9(3):1-6.

28. Ziskin MC, Petitti DB. Epidemiology of human exposure to ultrasound: a critical review. *Ultrasound Med Biol.* 1988;14(2):91-96.

29. Lyons EA, Dyke C, Toms M, Cheang M, Math M. In utero exposure to diagnostic ultrasound: a 6-year follow-up. *Radiology.* 1988;166:687-690.

30. Stark CR, Orleans M, Haverkamp AD, Murphy J. Short- and long-term risks after exposure to diagnostic ultrasound in utero. *Obstet Gynecol.* 1984; 63:194-200.

31. Hellman LM, Duffus GM, Donald I, Sunden B. Safety of diagnostic ultrasound in obstetrics. *Lancet.* 1970;1:1133-1135.

32. Scheidt PD, Stanley F, Bryla DA: One year follow-up of infants exposed to ultrasound in utero. *Am J Obstet Gynecol.* 1978;113:2119-2121.

33. Bakketeig LS, Eik-Nes SH, Jacobsen G, Ulstein MK, Brodtkorb CJ, Balstad P, Ericksen BC, Jorgensen NP: A randomized controlled trial of ultrasonographic screening in pregnancy. *Lancet.* 1984;2:207-210.

34. Cartwright RA, McKinney PA, Hopton PA, Birch JM, Hartley Al, Mann JR, et al. Ultrasound examinations in pregnancy and childhood cancer. *Lancet.* 1984;2:999-1000.

35. Kinnier-Wilson, Waterhouse JA. Obstetrical ultrasound and childhood malignancies. *Lancet.* 1984;2:997-999.

36. David H, Weaver JB, Pearson JF. Doppler ultrasound and fetal activity. *Br Med J.* 1975;2:62-64.

37. Hertz RH, Timor-Tritsch I, Dierker LJ, Chik L, Rosen MG. Continuous ultrasound and fetal movements. *Am J Obstet Gynecol.* 1979;135:152-154.

38. Powell-Phillips WD, Towell ME. Doppler ultrasound and subjective assessment of fetal activity. *Br Med J.* 1979;2:101-102.

39. Saint-Anne Dargassies S. *The Neuro-Motor and Psycho-Affective Development of the Infant.* New York, NY: Elsevier; 1986.

40. Mole R. Possible hazards of imaging and doppler ultrasound in obstetrics. *Birth.* 1986;13:23-32.

41. Meire HB. The safety of diagnostic ultrasound. *Br J Obstet Gynecol.* 1987;94:1121-1122.

42. British Institute of Radiology. The safety of diagnostic ultrasound. Report of the Royal College of Obstetricians and Gynecologists; 1987.

43. Sparling JW, Wilhelm IJ, MacLeod AM, Green S, Katz V, Huntington GS, Blanchard G, Aydlett L. Developing a taxonomy of fetal movement: the first step in a longitudinal collaborative study. *Phys Occup Ther Pediatr.* 1990;10:43-46.

44. Folio MR, Fewell RR. *Peabody Developmental Motor Scales and Activity Cards.* Allen, TX: DLM Teaching Resources; 1983.

45. Howell DC. *Statistical Methods for Psychology.* Boston, MA: Duxbury Press; 1982.

46. Thun-Hohenstein L, Largo RH, Molinari L, Kundu S, Duc G. Early fine motor and adaptive development in high-risk appropriate for gestational age preterm and healthy term children. *Eur J Pediatr.* 1991;150:562-569.

47. Forslund M, Bjerre I. Follow-up of preterm children. II.growth and development at four years of age. *Early Hum Dev.* 1990;24:107-118.

48. Largo RH, Molinari L, Kundu S, Hunziker U, Duc G. Neurological outcome in high-risk weight appropriate for gestational age preterm children at early school age. *Eur J Pediatr.* 1990;149:835-844.

49. Cohen SE, Parmelee AH, Beckwith L, Sigman M. Cognitive development in preterm births:birth to 8 years. *J Dev Behav Pediatr.* 1986;7(2):102-110.

50. Friedman SL, Jacobs BS, Werthmann MW. Preterms of low medical risk: spontaneous behaviors and soothability at expected date of birth. *Infant Behavior and Development.* 1982;5:3-10.

51. Miller LJ. Miller Assessment for Preschoolers. San Antonio, TX: Psychological Corporation; 1988.

Quantitative Measurement
of Fetal Movement:
Fetal-Posture and Movement Assessment
(F-PAM)

Joyce W. Sparling
Irma J. Wilhelm

SUMMARY. The history of quantitative measurement of fetal movement is reviewed, and problems with achieving reliability using ultrasound imaging for visualizing the fetus are discussed. Based on these factors, the seven phase process of developing a quantitative assessment of fetal movement is presented. The Fetal-Posture and Movement (F-PAM) system includes 20 categories emphasizing fetal posture and activity of the trunk and head, leg movement in space or against the uterine wall, arm movement towards specific objects, and jaw movements. The establishment of reliability and future directions for development and use of the assessment are suggested.

In the quantitative tradition, assessment is made of things as they are, independent of surrounding events or circumstances, and separate from interpretation.[1] Performing under this rationalistic perspective, investigators attempt to measure as objectively and precisely as possible. Standardized instrumentation and control are the foundation of the approach. Reliability, internal validity, and objectivity are the essential hallmarks implying the truthfulness of the measurements. Researchers asking quantitative questions try to "match statements to actual conditions."[1,p10] In exercising the quantitative perspective, investigators use a "neutral scientific or value-free language"[1,p11] to describe behavior.

This work has been supported in part by the Maternal and Child Health Postgraduate Training Grant 149, Department of Health and Human Services.

The purpose of this paper is to present a quantitative instrument for describing fetal movement. Once systematic development is completed, the instrument may be used for measuring the activity of the developing fetus in order to support qualitative assessment, augment other quantitative measures, and answer specific finite rather than interpretive research questions.

BACKGROUND

The measurement of human fetal movement has been a relatively uncharted area of investigation, with problems of reliability and validity accompanying all measurement attempts. Some of these problems emanate from asking questions about three-dimensional motion from two-dimensional schema, such as ultrasound imaging of movement, and even maternal perception of movement. For centuries, the only way to measure fetal movement was by maternal perception. This methodology persists, but recent studies have shown its limitations. Not only do pregnant women not sense movements until 17-21 weeks of gestation, but mothers perceive 27-75 percent fewer movements than observed on ultrasound scan,[2] and have difficulty differentiating general movements from isolated limb movements.[3, 4] These limitations prevent establishing reliability with this form of measurement. More valid and reliable measurement methods are needed to describe the variability and development of fetal movement.

Types of Quantitative Assessment

Equipment. The history of the quantitative measurement of fetal movement is interwoven with the development of various types of technology. Preyer[5] first used auscultation via a stethoscope to detect movement. Twenty years later the kymograph was placed on the mother's abdomen to detect changes in abdominal contour resulting from underlying fetal movements.[6] Pressure sensitive external monitoring devices, such as the tocodynamometer[7] have been used because they permit non-invasive assessment of gross fetal movements, and have no energy interaction with the patient, unlike ultrasound.[8] B-mode linear ultrasound scans[9,10] allow real-time assessment of fetal movement and improved views of specific parts of the fetal anatomy.

Besides the question of safety, a number of limitations accompany the use of ultrasound and complicate the valid and reliable collection of data. Observing and recording fetal movements via real-time ultrasound are labor-intensive, and error rates are highly variable because of the changing planes and periodicities of fetal movements. Sector scans can distort the fetal image by showing different depths of fields, and varying magnifications can be set as defaults on different machines, thus modifying the investigator's focus on parts or whole body actions. The internal calibration of the machines is not equal to external measuring devices requiring careful checks and corrections. Safety has also been questioned, as described in the Tucker et al. article in this issue, although no definitive research supports any danger of its use with humans.

One controversial perspective associated with the use of ultrasound is the contention that the pulsed soundwaves themselves stimulate fetal activity thus invalidating the assessment of spontaneous movement. In 1975, a group of Welsh researchers[11] used 45 minutes of imaging with 36 patients and determined that a mean increase in fetal activity of over 90 percent occurred with Doppler imaging. Fetal activity was determined with subjective ratings by the maternal subject. Several years later a group of Scottish researchers[12] suggested that the way fetal movements had been counted in that study was unclear and that in their controlled study they found no effect of Doppler ultrasound on movement.

Three-dimensional (3-D) ultrasound is now technically possible. Its clinical use is imminent and will greatly enhance measurement of fetal movement. 3-D technology will permit differentiation of movement characteristics at various gestational ages and among a wide variety of diagnostic groups. Coding systems that are exhaustive and have independent categories will be valued adjuncts to assessment using 3-D technology.

Fetal Movement Behavioral Assessments. Observation of human fetal movement has been wedded to the technology of real-time ultrasound since its early use in the 1970's. One of the earliest investigators using real-time ultrasound,[13] assessed the number of movements in a five-minute scan and revealed that "brisk" movements occurred 4-9 times/minute and "slow, sluggish" movements occurred 1-4 times/minute in pregnancies determined to be within normal limits. Other early ultrasound researchers[14] used 30-second to 5-minute gray scale imagings with a mean power output of 10 mW/cm^2 to study 37 women. They identified nine movements, from twitch occurring at 7 weeks, to locomotor movements of arms and legs at 15 weeks, to periodic repetitive movements of the diaphragm at 27 weeks. In a brief paper, these investigators described many of the problems of fetal movement assessment, yet remained enthusiastic about its future directions.

Another type of quantitative assessment of movement has been developed by obstetricians. The Biophysical Profile[15] is a clinical scale that includes five parameters of fetal breathing movements, body movements, tone, amniotic fluid volume, and heart rate reactivity. Each of these parameters is given a score of 0-2. A total score of 8-10 is regarded as normal for a fetus. In scoring "gross body movement" over the 30-minute period, the presence of three or more discrete body or limb movements is designated as "normal," while two or fewer episodes of body/limb movements in this time period denote abnormal behavior. Several problems exist for this approach. Thirty minutes of imaging is not allowed by some human subject review boards in the United States and Canada. In addition, the one to two cm rule for determining normal amounts of fluid is a subjective designation, and heart rates vary at different gestational ages and under varying normal conditions. Although such gross assessment is not sufficient to distinguish subtleties of movement, other methods have been developed that might differentiate fetuses according to neuromuscular status.

The most definitive quantitative assessments of fetal movement have come from Prechtl's laboratory.[16-19] Judgments were made of real-time fetal movement using hand-activated event markers and a pre-established coding scheme including 16 movements. The movements have been identified and an actogram depicting their presence and order of appearance has been used with the 7 to 19 week fetus.[20] General movements are defined as "gross movements involving the whole body. They may last from a few seconds to a minute. . . . They wax and wane in intensity, force and speed, and their onset and end are gradual. The majority of extension or flexion of arms and legs is complex, with superimposed rotations and often slight changes in direction of the movement. . . . the movement is fluent and elegant and creates the impression of complexity and variability."[21,p152-153] The intricacy of these movements appears to have led these researchers to the designation of "general" movements as the most meaningful fetal motor behavior[21] and the ones that should be assessed for frequency and duration.[16,17,19]

Jorgensen et al.[22] used two linear array real-time ultrasound imagers and a time-distance recorder to determine the number of movements during a 30-minute segment. For 10-, 11-, and 12-week fetuses, 150 to 159 movements occurred at each age. If this assessment is accurate, then the validity of the Biophysical Profile must be questioned in that it requires observation of three movements per 30-minute segment for a "normal" evaluation. Further study with Jorgensen et al.'s approach is being conducted to evaluate the effect of drugs on fetal movements and to try and give some meaning to these numbers.

These approaches to measuring fetal movement all have some validity. All have been hampered, however, by the use of two-dimensional rather than three-dimensional ultrasound. The reliability of human observations of two-dimensional images continues to be problematic.

Reliability

Several methods of achieving reliability of fetal movement assessment have been described. Prechtl's group has used consensus of six to ten obstetricians viewing videotaped segments of real-time images. In one report, ten physicians achieved an "average percentage of agreement"[21,p155] of 90 percent (range 75-100) on assessment of 10 normal and 10 abnormal fetuses. These observers were challenged to label preselected segments of "general movements" as normal or abnormal. The reliability of a similar diagnostic judgment was 89 percent by eight observers of five growth-retarded and five non-growth-retarded fetuses.[17] To achieve this figure, the number of "general movements" occurring in 40-second episodes was scored.

The Delphi group opinion method[23] has been used by Swartjes et al.[24] and vanWoerden et al.[25] to enable groups of investigators to come to some agreement on their observations of fetal movements. Through several rounds of anonymous scoring of observations, followed by controlled feedback of the results from the previous scoring, and statistical report of the group's scoring, the group comes to a consensus on the observations. The larger the group, the greater the accuracy and the higher the reliability. In the first round of scoring of four behaviors in the vanWoerden et al. study, the three observers disagreed 19.4 percent of the total time scoring was conducted. In the second round, this percent decreased to 10.7. In the final round, 6.1 percent of the imaging was unable to be classified, and in 2.7 percent no agreement could be reached. Other groups have rescored a small percentage of the total recordings to determine reliability of the data. Roodenburg et al.[18] rescored four percent of the original tapes and obtained a 1.6 to 2.2 percent standard deviation of the scores of two observers. The variety of approaches to reliability reflects the difficulty in scoring complex movement and suggests the need for more precise measurement systems that include an exhaustive and independent set of motor behaviors.

METHODOLOGY

Subjects

Over a period of one year, 20 women experiencing a low-risk pregnancy were identified from the private obstetric clinic at a tertiary care hospital. Their mean age was 28.7 years, the mean grade level completed was 17.5 and their occupations placed them in the highest two categories of Hollingshead's socioeconomic categories.[26] The first fetus of these maternal subjects was nonviable. Videotapes of the next two were made every two weeks until 20 weeks, and thereafter every 5 weeks until 35 weeks of pregnancy. Of the next subgroup of 12 subjects, one subject was not pregnant, and one subject spontaneously aborted at 35 weeks. The remaining subjects were identified by 12 weeks, and videotaped at 12, 14, 16, and 18 weeks. Four additional subjects were assessed every two weeks from 12 to 18 weeks and agreed to have their infant assessed at birth with the Brazelton Neonatal Behavioral Assessment Scale.[27] Over 40 hours of ultrasound scans of these subjects, observed at 100 frames-per-second, provided the data for the development of our assessment instrument, the Fetal-Posture and Movement System (F-PAM).

Instrumentation

A 3.5 MHx linear array ultrasound with 1/2″ videotape recorder was used for imaging. Scoring of the videotaped images was assisted with direct data entry using The Observational Coding System (OCS),[28] a software package designed for this purpose. With this software package, time codes can be overlaid on the tape and synchronized with the computer entry file. In addition, the file of scores can be overlaid on the videotape enabling easy data editing on replay of scored segments. The OCS permits merging of at least five separately coded data sets, so is amenable to complex data manipulation.

Four physical therapists experienced in assessing movement of preterm and full term infants acted as raters. These raters had viewed at least 100 hours of ultrasound imagings prior to scoring these videotapes.

Procedure

Phase 1. The literature pertaining to fetal movement was reviewed and measurement tools used to record movement were evaluated. Through consultation with a computer programmer, the Observational Coding System was determined to be the software most consistent with our observational assessment needs of overlay and merging.[29]

Phase 2. An interdisciplinary team of investigators was identified. Consent was obtained to videotape the ultrasound imagings of 20 subjects from 10 to 16 weeks of gestation. Movements of the mothers' fetuses were filmed every 14 days from 12 to 20 weeks and at 25, 30 and 35 weeks. Maintaining a systems perspective, we interviewed the mothers to evaluate their pregnancy experience and to remain informed on the progression of the pregnancy.[30]

Phase 3. Throughout the development process, three videotapes were randomly selected for intensive study during each phase of the project. The first group of three 30-minute videotaped imagings of fetal subjects at 12, 14 and 16 weeks of gestation were observed frame-by-frame by two physical therapists. A 100 frames-per-second time code was superimposed on the tapes which were run in four different modes in order to identify movements. The tapes were first observed real-time, then frame-by-frame, and, where helpful, were run fast forward and fast reverse. Over 75 hours of observation permitted the determination of active and inactive periods, and symmetry and asymmetry of movements during the active and inactive periods at each gestational age. Judgment was by consensus.

Results of this first phase and a videotape of typical arm movements were presented at a Pediatric Combined Sections meeting of the American Physical Therapy Association.[31] The results indicated: a greater amount of activity relative to inactivity at 14 weeks than at any other time; an increase in activity from 12 to 14 weeks and a decrease in activity from 14 to 16 weeks; no differences in the amount of time that the arms were symmetrical or asymmetrical; but more asymmetry during active periods than during inactive periods (Table 1). These preliminary results led directly to establishing an inductive methodology for developing a tool for more accurately measuring these apparent changes.

Phase 4. Recognizing the need for both qualitative and quantitative measurement,[1] two teams were established, one to use an inductive, and one a deductive, approach to assessment development. The deductive approach is described by Green and Sparling in this issue. The inductive approach is the focus of this paper.

The inductive approach was used to observe in a relatively unbiased fashion what was occurring in three additional fetal videotapes at 12, 14 and 16 weeks. Prior to scoring specific movements, three preliminary descriptions of the imagings were required: the segments of tape that were clear and able to be scored were noted and the exact times of usable tape were entered into the computer; the view of the fetus was described, e.g., sagittal or frontal; and the position of the fetus relative to gravity was recorded where possible. These designations are shown in Figure 1.

Because much of the observed movement was related to the

Table 1 - Percent of Usable Tape in which Symmetrical and Asymmetrical Arm Movements Occur during Active and Inactive Periods for Three Fetuses at 12, 14 and 16 Weeks of Gestation

Periods	Subjects								
	1	2	3	1	2	3	1	2	3
	(12 weeks GA)			(14 weeks GA)			(16 weeks GA)		
Inactivity	55	49	60	30	09	19	23	54	44
Activity	45	51	40	70	91	81	77	46	56
Asymmetry	54	71	52	46	62	44	42	36	04
Symmetry	46	29	48	54	38	56	58	64	96
Asymmetry	13	78	22	58	22	75	56	100	53
Symmetry/ Inactivity	87	22	78	42	78	25	44	00	47
Aymmetry	87	91	100	70	100	00	100	100	100
Symmetry/ Activity	13	09	00	30	00	100	00	00	00

trunk, that became the first body category to be described (Figure 2). A large number of body movements appeared to be related to cervical movement, so the head and neck movements were next recorded (Figure 3). Sections on right and left leg movements were developed, and a third category on legs was added when the plane of observation did not permit certainty about which leg was being observed (Figure 4). A major characteristic of the legs were their use of the uterine wall during inactive and active periods, a characteristic requiring a category for describing the legs in contact with the wall or in space. Scoring of arm movements was complicated by the apparent directionality of the movements. The directional component of the arm movements led to an additional designation for the arms categories of direction of movement, followed by location of movement in terms of body quadrants (Figure 5). From our earlier observations, the fetus was either inactive or active, therefore categories of posture as well as movement, were designated for

Figure 1 - Categories 1, 2 and 3 of the Fetal-Posture and
Movement (F-PAM) System

1. QUALITY OF IMAGING FOR SCORING

    1-0 Not usable
    1-1 Usable for total body
    1-2 Usable only for upper body
    1-3 Usable only for lower body

2. VIEW

    2-0 Not usable/can't score
    2-1 Caudal
    2-2 Coronal
    2-3 Dorsal
    2-4 Ventral
    2-5 Sagittal
    2-6 Ventral/coronal

2-2 - Coronal View

3. POSITION IN RELATION TO GRAVITY

3-00 Not usable/can't score
(14 positions are depicted for ventral and sagittal views)

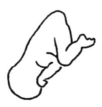

Sagittal View - 3-07 Head down, trunk diagonal, prone

Figure 2 - Categories 4 and 5 of the Fetal-Posture and
         Movement (F-PAM) System

4. AMOUNT/DEGREE OF TRUNK MOVEMENT

4-0 Not usable/can't score
4-1 Small-<20° from start
4-2 Moderate-20-80°
4-3 Large->80°
4-4 No movement

5. TRUNK POSTURE AND MOVEMENT

5-00 Not usable/can't score
(17 positions are depicted for ventral and sagittal views)
5-05 given as example

Sagittal view - Trunk Posture Flexed

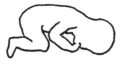

each body part. This initial classification scheme was presented for feedback at a national physical therapy conference.[32]

Phase 5. Preparations for a content analysis of the instrument permitted further clarification of leg movements and addition of mouth movements. A content analysis was conducted with four physical therapy assessment experts who were unfamiliar with the analysis of fetal movement.[33] After a brief training period, they observed the 20 categories of movement, scored each one and then rated each section on independence, and the whole instrument on comprehensiveness. Although a more intensive content analysis will be conducted, these movement experts with relative ease identified selected behaviors according to our categories.

Phase 6. Based on this feedback, problem areas were clarified. Dorsal views were eliminated and only sagittal and ventral views were included for scoring. For example, leg abduction could not be scored from the sagittal view, just as leg flexion could not be scored from a dorsal view. A protocol for scoring the videotapes of fetal

Figure 3 - Categories Categories 6 and 7 of the Fetal-
Posture and Movement (F-PAM) System

6. AMOUNT/DEGREE OF HEAD MOVEMENT

6-0 Not usable/can't score
6-1 Small-<20° from start
6-2 Moderate-20-80°
6-3 Large->80°
6-4 No movement

7. HEAD POSTURE AND MOVEMENT

(15 positions are depicted for ventral and sagittal views)
7-11 given as example

Ventral view - Head rotated left

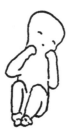

imagings was completed and a random selection of 31, one-minute segments of tape were selected and scored independently by the authors. A "confusion matrix"[34] was established based on this data.

Phase 7. The discriminant validity of the F-PAM is presently being conducted with a sample of fetuses exposed to cocaine, and another study is planned with fetuses of diabetic women. In addition, specific movements will be merged to systematically determine the development of patterns of movement.

RESULTS

The Fetal-Posture and Movement (F-PAM) system is a 20-item research instrument developed to assess spontaneous fetal move-

Figure 4 - Categories 8-13 of the Fetal-Posture and Movement
           (F-PAM) System

8. AMOUNT/LOCATION OF RIGHT LOWER EXTREMITY

    8-0 Not usable/can't score
    8-1 Small-<20° from start
    8-2 Moderate-20-80°
    8-3 Large->80°
    8-4 No movement

11. RIGHT LEG POSTURE AND MOVEMENT

(14 positions are depicted for ventral and sagittal views)
        11-050711-05 given as example

Ventral View - Hip flexed (05), abducted (07), externally
rotated (11), knee flexed (05)

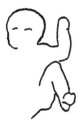

ment. The first three sections of the instrument are described in
Figure 1. These sections must be scored prior to scoring either with
the F-PAM or the deductively derived assessment, the Q-MOVE,
described in this issue. A file is established of these three categories
for each videotape, enabling researchers to quickly access usable
sections of tape, saving countless hours of perusing tapes for appropriate sections for studying a specific body segment. In addition,
reliability on the movements will be enhanced if these preliminary
decisions have already been made.

The next 17 categories include posture and movement and are
described in Figures 2 through 5. Several examples are given for
clarification. For each body part, posture or amount and kind of
movement are described. Sample scores for each example are included.

Figure 5 - Categories 14-19 of the Fetal-Posture and
            Movement (F-PAM) System

15. AMOUNT OF LEFT UPPER EXTREMITY MOVEMENT

        15-0 Not usable/can't score
        15-1 Small-<20° from start
        15-2 Moderate-20-80°
        15-3 Large->80°
        15-4 No movement

18. LEFT ARM POSTURE AND MOVEMENT

(21 directions of movement and 36 locations of movement)
    are depicted for ventral and sagittal views
            18-2-01-05 given as example

18 (left arm), 1 (movement), 01 (perioral region), 05
    (quadrant 1 to upper midline)

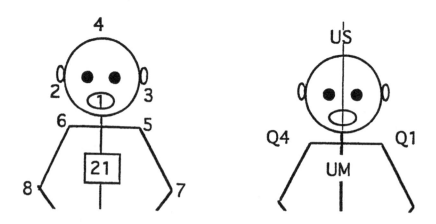

Interrater reliability ranged from 33 to 85 percent depending on a number of factors, especially the number of decisions that had to be made to obtain a score. In some cases this process consisted of 15 decisions for one score because the raters were scoring all 20 categories.

DISCUSSION

Reliable and valid measurement requires the use of systematically developed assessment instruments.[35, 36] Based on factors described for developing an observational coding system,[34] we inductively formulated the F-PAM and are in the process of achieving reliability using it. Determination of interrater reliability is an elusive process. Because we tried to obtain reliability on all 20 categories of movement, we did not always achieve an acceptable interrater reliability. We suggest that training and scoring on the posture and movement of the head, or trunk, or upper or lower extremities is indicated to achieve consistently acceptable reliability. For training purposes, a confusion matrix[34] can be established to assist with training and to compute a Cohen's kappa. In the authors' scoring of a random sample of the first three categories of the F-PAM, categories in which we were consistently unreliable were noted and the assessment modified accordingly. For example, the first observer scored ventral view (4) while the second observer scored ventral-coronal (6) (Figure 1).

We are discussing the development of the instrument at this time to elicit the support of other investigators in the process of determining the validity and reliability of the tool. In addition, as more investigators become involved in the measurement of fetal movement, use of the same criteria for scoring movements will facilitate the development of a data bank. The need for a larger subject pool is particularly important if we are to make pronouncements about the developing nervous system through our study of fetal movement.

Much of fetal movement assessment to date has been qualitative, with Prechtl[21] declaring that qualitative assessment using Gestalt perception is the most meaningful. Many attempts are being made to quantify those qualitative assessments, and to fuse effectively these two approaches to measurement. These attempts appear to be inconsistent with the position of Smith and Heshusius[1] that the two approaches are, indeed, different and that the use of either approach is dependent on the question asked. The questions that may be posited related to this area of research are legion:

1. Can individual patterns of fetal motor development be identified that would help direct our study of the sensorimotor development of a child?

2. Are discrete fetal movements coordinated into motor patterns? Once developed, are these patterns repeated? Are preprogrammed movements a component of motor development?
3. Do early patterns of movement relate to later functional activity, e.g., crawling, walking?
4. What occurs in the impaired developing fetus: a regression to earlier motor patterns;[37,38] or a change in the amount, frequency or duration of movements; or a delay in the appearance of movements?
5. Do fetal and neonatal movements have continuity, e.g., is pedalling by the fetus the precursor to the discontinuous stepping pattern of the neonate?
6. Can we use acoustic stimulation as a treatment for motor delay in utero?

CONCLUSION

The potential for understanding motor development from its inception is now a reality. Observable movement starts at least by seven weeks of gestation and is modified by environmental as well as endogenous factors. Visualization of the fetus has enabled investigators to describe movements and to correlate their presence with other physiologic changes, such as breathing movements, eye movements and heart rate changes. Through continued study of early fetal movement with more precise measurements, we may clarify the relationship of early movements to functional activity and help explain the transition from the fetal to neonatal period. We may thereby gain a deeper understanding of the behavior of preterm infants and of fetuses experiencing impaired motor development and prepare for prenatal intervention.

REFERENCES

1. Smith JK, Heshusius L. Closing down the conversation: the end of the quantitative-qualitative debate among educational inquirers. *Educ Research.* 1986; 15(1):4-12.

2. Kisilevsky BS, Killen H, Muir DW, Low JA. Maternal and ultrasound measurements of elicited fetal movements: a methodologic consideration. *Obstet Gynecol.* 1991;77:889-892.

3. Gettinger A, Roberts AB, Campbell S. Comparison between subjective and ultrasound assessments of fetal movement. *Br Med J.* 1978;2:88-90.

4. Hertogs K, Roberts AB, Cooper D, Griffin DR, Campbell S. Maternal perception of fetal motor activity. *Br Med J.* 1979;22:1183-1185.

5. Preyer W: *Spezielle Physiologie des Embryo.* Leipzig, Gaareiben: 1985.

6. Tuck SM. Ultrasound monitoring of fetal behaviour. *Ultrasound Med Biol.* 1986;12(4):307-317.

7. Timor-Tritsch I, Zador I, Hertz RH, Rosen MG. Classification of human fetal movement. *Am J Obstet Gynecol.* 1976;126:70-77.

8. Sorokin Y, Pillay S, Dierker LJ, Hertz RH, Rosen MG. A comparison between maternal, tocodynamometric, and real-time ultrsonographic assessments of fetal movement. *Am J Obstet Gynecol.* 1981;140:456-460.

9. Hoffman D, Hollander HJ. On the detection of fetal life and the measurement of the child's skull by means of two-dimensional ultrasonic echo process. *Gynaecologia.* 1968;165:60-61.

10. Seeds JW, Cefalo RC. *Practical Obstetrical Ultrasound.* Rockville, MD: Aspen Publishers; 1986.

11. David H, Weaver JB, Pearson JF. Doppler ultrasound and fetal activity. *Br Med J.* 1975;2:62-64.

12. Phillips WDP, Towell ME. Doppler ultrasound and subjective assessment of fetal activity. *Br Med J.* 1979;July 14:101-102.

13. Reinold E. Ultrasonics in early pregnancy. *Contrib Gynecol Obstet.* 1976; 1:102-127.

14. Birnholz JC, Stephens JC, Faria M. Fetal movement patterns: a possible means of defining neurologic developmental milestones in utero. *Am J Roentgenol.* 1978; 130:537-540.

15. Manning FA, Platt LD, Sipos L. Antepartum fetal evaluation: development of a biophysical profile. *Am J Obstet Gynecol.* 1980;136:787-795.

16. deVries JIP, Visser GHA, Prechtl HFR. The emergence of fetal behaviour. II. quantitative aspects. *Early Hum Dev.* 1985;12:99-120.

17. Bekedam DJ, Visser GHA, deVries JJ, Prechtl HFR. Motor behaviour in the growth retarded fetus. *Early Hum Dev.* 12:155-165, 1985.

18. Roodenburg PJ, Wladimiroff JW, vanEs A, Prechtl HFR. Classification and quantitative aspects of fetal movements during the second half of normal pregnancy. *Early Hum Dev.* 1991;25:19-35.

19. Visser GHA, Laurini RN, deVries JIP, Bekedam DJ, Prechtl HFR. Abnormal motor behaviour in anencephalic fetuses. *Early Hum Dev.* 1985;12:173-182.

20. deVries JIP, Visser GHA, Prechtl HFR. The emergence of fetal behaviour. I.qualitative aspects. *Early Hum Dev.* 1982;7:301-322.

21. Prechtl HFR. Qualitative changes of spontaneous movements in fetus and preterm infant are a marker of neurological dysfunction. *Early Hum Dev.* 1990; 23:151-158.

22. Jorgensen NP, Marsal K, Lindstrom K. Quantification of fetal motor activity in early pregnancy. *Eur J Obstet Gynecol Reprod Biol.* 1989;30:11-18.

23. Dalkey N. An experimental study of group opinion: the Delphi method. *Futures.* 1969:408-426.

24. Swartjes JM, vanGeijn HP, Meinardi H, vanAlphen M, Schoemaker HC. Fetal rest-activity cycles and chronic exposure to antiepileptic drugs. *Epilepsia.* 1991;32(5):722-728.

25. vanWoerden EE, vanGeijn HP, Caron FJM, Swartjes JM, Mantel R, Arts NFTh. Automated assignment of behavioral states in the human near term fetus. *Early Hum Dev.* 1989;19:137-146.

26. Hollingshead's Two-Factor Index. New Haven, CT.

27. Brazelton TB. *Neonatal Behavioral Assessment Scale, 2nd ed. Clinics in Developmental Medicine* 88. Philadelphia, PA: JB Lippincott; 1984.

28. Szostek TK. *Observational Coding System.* Research Triangle Park, NC: Research Triangle Collaborative;1988.

29. Sparling J. Observational research using the automated coding system, abstracted. *Phys Ther.* 1988;68:865.

30. Sparling JW, Wilhelm IJ, MacLeod AM, Green SD, Katz VL, Blanchard GF, Huntington GS, Aydlett LA. Developing a taxonomy of fetal movement: the first step in a longitudinal collaborative study. *Phys Occup Ther Pediatr.* 1990; 10(1):43-46.

31. Sparling JW, Wilhelm IJ. The qualitative assessment of fetal arm movements, abstracted. *Phys Ther.* 1989;69:397.

32. Sparling JW, Wilhelm IJ, Katz VL. A taxonomy of fetal movement. Poster presented at the Combined Sections Meeting, APTA, New Orleans, LA: February 3, 1990.

33. Sparling JW, Wilhelm IJ. The content validity of the Fetal Movement Classification System. Paper presented at the Second Annual Maternal and Child Health Leadership Conference, Chicago, Ill: April, 1990.

34. Bakeman R, Gottman JM. *Observing Interaction: An introduction to Sequential Analysis.* New York, NY: Cambridge University Press;1989.

35. Wilhelm IJ, ed. *Physical Therapy Assessment in Early Infancy.* New York, NY: Churchill Livingstone; 1992.

36. Miller LJ, ed. *Developing Norm-referenced Standardized Tests.* New York, NY: Haworth Press; 1989.

37. Ianniruberto A, Tajani E. Ultrasonic study of fetal movements. *Semin Perinatol.* 1981;5:175-181.

38. Milani Comparetti A. Pattern analysis of normal and abnormal development: The fetus, the newborn, the child. In: Slaton D, ed: *Development of Movement in Infancy.* Chapel Hill, NC: University of North Carolina; 1980.

Q-MOVE:
Development of a Qualitative Assessment of Fetal Movement

Sandra Green
Joyce W. Sparling

SUMMARY. The study of fetal movement has been characterized in qualitative and quantitative ways. This paper clarifies the use of the term "qualitative" and describes previously developed qualitative assessments of movement. Based on Laban's, Kestenberg's and Al's theories of movement analysis and their terminology, the process of developing a qualitative scale to assess fetal movement is described. The components of the instrument are presented and future use of the research tool are suggested.

Normal human fetal movement, spontaneous and reflexive, is observed at 7.5 weeks gestational age (GA). Coordination of movements into identifiable patterns occurs at least by 15-20 weeks gestational age.[1,2] Qualitative differences in these complex, spontaneous

Sandra Green completed her entry-level physical therapy training at the University of North Carolina at Chapel Hill and is now affiliated with a clinical site in Pittsboro, NC. Joyce W. Sparling, PhD, PT, OT, is Assistant Professor in the Division of Physical Therapy at the University of North Carolina at Chapel Hill. She is Project Director for the Maternal and Child Health Postgraduate Training Grant.

This work was supported in part by an Innovative Research Award from the Frank Porter Graham Research and Child Development Center, a Department of Medical Allied Health Professions Starter Grant, and a Maternal and Child Health Bureau Postgraduate Training Grant from the Department of Health and Human Services.

For additional information regarding the Q-MOVE Manual and training opportunities, please contact the authors at CB #7135, Wing E, University of North Carolina at Chapel Hill, Chapel Hill, NC 27599-7135.

115

fetal movements have been used as indicators of neurological status.[3, 4] The most sensitive indicators of neural integrity, accortading to Prechtl, are gross "general" movements involving the whole body. General movements in the normal healthy fetus are "fluent and elegant," creating an "impression of complexity and variability."[3,p153]

The subtle underlying kinetic components of complex spontaneous fetal movements have received limited examination because of the lack of adequate motor assessments and the two-dimensional nature of images. The purpose of this paper is to describe the systematic process of developing a theory-based movement assessment designed to differentiate the qualitative characteristics of early human movement. Our analysis differs from previous fetal movement research in its deductive application of a movement analysis system to organize observations. The result of this approach is the Qualitative Assessment of Fetal Movement (Q-MOVE). In this paper, movement quality is defined, previous work on assessing fetal motor quality is reviewed, and four movement analysis systems are described. One of these systems is applied to the formation of the Q-MOVE.

MOVEMENT QUALITY

The quality of a motion is the *way* in which a movement takes place, the "how" or style of a movement. Any movement or sequence of movements may be expressed in a variety of ways. Quality refers to the simultaneous blending of characteristics of spatial use, time and force quality into dynamic patterns of movement. In contrast to qualitative analysis and its focus on movement style and dynamics, quantitative analysis addresses the objective characteristics of motor activities that may include frequency, duration, velocity and amplitude. Both types of analysis offer a critical perspective on fetal movement and health status.

In quantitative studies, the frequency of fetal movement has been related typically to heart rate variations,[7] behavioral states,[8] and circadian sleep-activity cycles.[9] Accurate visualization of the fetal movement is not always possible, however, preventing the achievement of adequate reliability in quantifying movement characteristics. For example, measuring force accurately is difficult when exact mass and velocity cannot be precisely determined. Although three-dimensional (3-D) ultrasound imaging will help with this problem, we are some years away from a commercially available 3-D imaging system. Qualitative assessment, however, permits evaluation of the subtle characteristics of fetal movement. An accurate recording system is needed to describe more reliably these subtle features of fetal motility.

History

The modern history of fetal movement assessment began with nineteenth century investigations of quickening, the time at which the mother first senses fetal movement. Fetal motility was known to exist, however, long before the mother's initial report of movement at 14-22 weeks of gestation.[8] In the late 1880's, Preyer used palpation and the stethoscope to detect this early movement and recognized even then its spontaneous nature.[9]

Contrary to the opinion of Preyer, Hooker[10] and Humphrey[11] believed fetal motility was mainly reflexive in origin. Although he knew of Preyer's work, Hooker thought that a primary phase of movement existed that resulted from exteroceptive stimulation. Movements in response to stimuli were characterized as stereotyped, patterned, identical and constant within the pattern. Hooker's and Humphrey's research was conducted on spontaneously aborted fetuses who survived only briefly outside of the uterus. Although they were primarily interested in identifying the onset of reflex movements, they did note that some movements seen at 8.5 and 9.5 weeks were spontaneous in nature. In addition, the quality of fetal response to stimulation changed from the automated and stereotyped movements seen at 8.5 weeks to smooth and fluid movements at 13.5 weeks.

The advent of ultrasound imaging permitted in utero observation of real-time movements. In 1978, Birnholz, Stephens, and Faria[12] conducted an ultrasound study based on Hooker's and Humphrey's categories of fetal movement. These investigators identified 11 movement patterns occurring between 6 and 40 weeks GA, but, in contrast to Hooker and Humphrey, described them as spontaneous.

The patterns were mainly denoted by body part and anatomical action. One category, "combined/repetitive," was similar to Prechtl's "general" movements and described "simultaneous or serial movements of the head or trunk and limbs which do not have a sudden, jerky or 'spastic' quality."

In one of the earliest real-time ultrasound studies of spontaneous fetal movement, Reinold[13] divided movements into two basic categories: strong, brisk movements or slow, sluggish movements. The strong movements had a forceful initial impulse involving the entire body and caused a change in fetal location and posture. No initial impulse was revealed with the slow movements, and only isolated body parts moved, with no change in trunk location or posture. Reinold observed a higher number of strong, brisk movements than slow, sluggish movements between 11 and 16 weeks GA in normal pregnancies and normal fetuses.

A more extensive ultrasound study was undertaken in 1981 by Ianniruberto and Tajani,[14] who followed 2000 subjects from 8-41 weeks of gestation. Their study specifically attempted to describe the quality of fetal movement patterns. In the conclusion of their study, the authors stated that fetal motor behavior was so "varied and rich" that their descriptions were "inadequate."[14,p180]

Milani Comparetti[15] applied the technique of "pattern analysis" developed with neonates and handicapped infants to the fetal data collected by Ianniruberto and Tajani. In this study, fetal movements were described as the primary motor patterns (PMP) that afford fetal locomotion, propulsive movements for birth, and other motor competencies necessary for survival. He concluded that no neonatal patterns originated at birth, since PMP's gave rise to all neonatal patterns. Milani Comparetti labelled actions as "propulsive" and used few qualitative descriptors to characterize the style of the movements.

The most extensive descriptions of the qualitative aspects of fetal movement have been provided by Ianniruberto and Tajani[14] and the deVries groups.[2] The longitudinal study by deVries, Visser and Prechtl[2] on the "emergence" and development of fetal movement contained details of action patterns and qualitative descriptors. The qualitative terminology used by these two groups is compared in Table 1. In comparing these two studies, every term referring to actions and action sequences was extracted from the two terminologies and organized according to use of space, time, and force.

Both groups describe the same fetal actions. The deVries group lists 16 patterns of movement corresponding to those seen by Ianniruberto and Tajani, with the addition of isolated retroflexion and anteflexion of the head. The deVries group, however, gives more detail of patterns, time usage, flow and initiation, but their assessment lacks description of the force of movements and some aspects of body shaping.

SYSTEMS OF MOVEMENT ANALYSIS

Movement analysis and notation systems have been applied to movement and movement behavior problems in dance, anthropology, ethology, behavioral psychology and physical education. The use of a movement analysis system provides methods or tools for data collection, recording and storage, and analysis. We reviewed four well-developed systems of analysis for possible application to fetal movement. All four include a two-dimensional symbolic notation system. Although they use entirely different descriptors, each system is organized, comprehensive and flexible.[16]

Laban Movement Analysis

The most comprehensive movement analysis system in wide use today is Laban Movement Analysis (LMA). Rudolf von Laban formulated his movement analysis theories in the early 1900's in Europe. Laban Movement Analysis and its related system, Effort-Shape Analysis, were developed by Laban,[17] a choreographer, Bartenieff,[18] a physical therapist, and researchers in the fields of dance, work motion analysis and psychology. Laban analysts view the body, in motion or at rest, in relation to the spatial context in which it moves; movement provides a means of interacting and coping with the environment.[18] LMA includes a symbol notation system used for choreographic notation and vocabulary for describing the essential movement qualities in categories of Effort and Shape. *Effort* terminology is descriptive of the force, speed, timing and

TABLE 1. Qualitative Terminology Used to Describe Fetal Movement by deVries, Visser, and Prechtl and by Ianniruberto and Tajani

	deVries, et al.	Ianniruberto & Tajani
Action words	startle, hiccup breathing movement, twitch, cloni, retro-flexion, jaw opening, stretch, yawn, ante-flexion extension, flexion, rotation	spasm, curling, jumps, startle, swallowing, expansion, retrac-tion, crossing, explore, thrust jerk, hiccup, scissoring, creep-ing, climbing, pulsating, opening closing, pedalling, floating extension, flexion, rotation
General qualitative adjectives	just-discernable, grace-ful, jerky, fluent	vermicular, jerky, smooth harmonious
Posture & shape	general, isolated, total alternating shifting contours	asymmetrical, amorphous, cephalic-caudal poles isolated, supine, prone, lateral, lying, symmetrical, reciprocal
Time	exact time of some move-ments given, rapid, slow, fast, prolonged, slow velocity, quick, abrupt, duration, higher speed, variable	rapid, quick, sudden, sluggish

Force of energy	amplitude, passive, forceful	vigorous
Flow & initiation	shifting of contours, one move leading to another, initiation in limbs-spreading to trunk, motion beginning in a place	jerks producing jumps, isolated segmental movement, rotation of trunk bringing about changes in position
Pattern	simultaneous, regular, repetitive, single event, rhythmical, irregular	simultaneous, rhythmic, sequence

coordinative qualities of movement and *Shape* describes the dynamic, changing configurations of trunk and limbs.

Kestenberg Movement Profile

The Kestenberg Movement Profile (KMP)[19,20] is a highly detailed system based on Effort-Shape and adapted for assessing the psychomotor function of infants and children. The KMP uses the flowing changes in body shape and locomotor patterns as indicators of personality development and parent-child interaction. The KMP also uses a graphic representation of movement, a flow diagram similar to an EKG recording. The diagram can be used to chart temporal and rhythm changes in motor activity.

Eshkohl-Wachmann System

The Eshkohl-Wachmann System[21] utilizes a geometric representation of joint movement. Limb movements and positions are described through an axial coordinate system, facilitating documentation of the trajectories of limb segments. The system has been used by Golani and Fentress[22] and Fentress[23] to describe developmental motor sequences in mice. The strength of the system lies in its capacity to describe fairly exact limb placement and pathways in space. The system does not describe movement qualities as does Effort-Shape Analysis nor does it support development of an action vocabulary.

Benesh Notation

LMA and its related system, Effort-Shape Analysis, and the Eshkohl-Wachmann System have been applied to problems of describing and recording human and animal motor behavior. A fourth system, Benesh Notation,[24] has been used by neurologists to document infant movement and the movements of handicapped children. In Benesh Notation, a five-line stave is used on which are superimposed symbols representing body parts and their position in space. Milani Comparetti and Gidoni[25] used the Benesh symbols to systematically notate movement. The Benesh system, unlike the LMA and its related Effort-Shape Analysis, is not based on a movement theory.

Because of the difficulty in observing real-time fetal movement and our interest in the qualitative aspects of movement, Effort-Shape Analysis was selected to guide the development of a more precise language to describe fetal movement. The Effort-Shape System permits analysis of movement in terms of space, force and time. In human movement, the body changes *shape,* often in relation to its environment, moving with some degree of *force,* over *time.*

METHODOLOGY

Subjects

Twenty pregnant women volunteered to participate in this study. They were evaluated as having a low-risk pregnancy by obstetricians at a tertiary care maternal and fetal medicine clinic. One subject was not pregnant and one fetus was nonviable. The mean age of the 18 remaining maternal subjects was 28.7 years, with a mean 17.5 years of education, describing a four-factor socioeconomic status (Hollingshead) of "1" or major professional for all but two subjects who were in category "3," clerical and sales work. All subjects experienced a normal pregnancy, were non-smokers, reported no use of drugs during their pregnancies, and were imaged at the same time of day from 4-6 PM. Procedures for identifying and obtaining videotaped images of the women's fetuses are described in the paper in this monograph by Sparling and Wilhelm. Fetuses ranged from 12-35 weeks gestational age, with all fetuses having images at 12, 14, 16, and 18 weeks of gestation.

Instrumentation

A 3.5 MHz linear array ultrasound scanner was used by a certified ultrasonographer to obtain the images. These images were copied on 1/2″ videotape, coded and stored for later blind scoring using a VCR, high resolution monitor and specially designed computer software.[26]

Two physical therapists (the authors) used Gestalt perception to observe the taped images and gain an overall sense of the dynamics of an action or action sequence. Gestalt perception has been used by Prechtl in analyzing fetal movements; it is an approach that "could not be replaced by automated quantification," and that Prechtl deemed appropriate for assessing complex phenomena such as fetal movement.[3,p154] The two observers applied anatomic and kinesiological knowledge, and observational and kinesthetic skills to differentiate movements and describe their qualities.

Procedure

The development of the Q-MOVE proceeded over a three-year period and consisted of five phases. The essential components of the Q-MOVE are shown in Table 2.

Phase 1: Effort Shape Analysis. Thirty-minute imagings of the fetal movements of 18 subjects at 12, 14, 16, and 18 weeks were conducted and videotaped for later observation. Videotapes of three of these ultrasound imagings were viewed to identify and critique the behaviors described by Ianniruberto and Tajani and deVries et al.

Table 2.   Qualitative Assessment of Fetal Movement (Q-MOVE)

BASIC MOVEMENT FACTORS

Spatial Use
Timing
Force Quality

DISCRETE ACTIONS AND ACTION SEQUENCES

Central Body Movements
Peripheral Body Movements
Action Sequences

ORGANIZATIONAL SUMMARY

Narrative
Flow Chart

Omissions and discrepancies in these two scales, when compared to the movement observed in the three imagings, led to a review of the Effort-Shape System for application to fetal movement assessment. From evaluation of these three videotapes and the Effort-Shape System, an initial formulation of Basic Movement Factors (BMF) was developed. BMF include the essential characteristics of movement: use of space, time, and force. The BMF data were presented for feedback by the senior author at a national physical therapy conference.[26]

Phase 2: Kestenberg Movement Profile Analysis. The Kestenberg Movement Profile (KMP) was used to help further delineate our descriptions. The senior author trained with Kestenberg and her associate, Sossin, in order to apply elements of the KMP to fetal movement (Personal instruction, October, 1989; January, 1990). Videotapes of two additional subjects at 12, 14, 16 and 18 weeks of gestation were reviewed because of their high motor content and excellent tape quality. Repeated analysis of the videotapes according to the KMP clarified aspects of shaping. Other KMP parameters were inadequate for delineating the timing and the force quality of the movements.

Kestenberg's flow diagram methodology was adapted for visually representing the flow of movement. A 30-second sample was selected from each of three tapes for observational analysis and graphic depiction of the flow of the observed movement. Approximately 20 viewings of the selected segment were necessary in order to create an accurate "flow diagram"[18] which captured minute changes in the gross activity of each fetus. Results of this approach using a 30-second segment of the tape are shown in Figures 1 and 2. A narrative "Impressions" of the whole 30-minute imaging is also presented. Subject 1 appeared to have an "organized" flow of movement and had a normal vaginal delivery at 40 weeks. Subject 3 appeared to have "disorganized" movement and spontaneously aborted at 35 weeks.

Phase 3: Time Sampling. The authors reviewed videotapes of three additional subjects at 12 and 14 weeks GA. These imagings were selected for gross differences among subjects in the amount of fetal movement, and were analyzed for characteristics of flow of motor activity, use of time, and body shaping. Analysis was con-

FIGURE 1. Narrative "Impression" of total 30-minute imaging and "Flow Diagram" of typical movement of Subject 1 at 14 weeks of gestation (from 15:50.00 to 16:20.00 minutes).

The 30-minute tape segment contained three clearly observable activity periods ranging from 1-5 minutes and four clearly observable rest periods from < 1-5.5 minutes. During rest and slow activity, the fetus was observed in a fetal tuck with the spine shaped to and supported by the uterine wall, and feet braced against the wall. During activity periods, all body segments moved in a wide variety of patterns of low to moderate force quality, moderate duration and with full use of space. Characteristic movements included: cervical to lumbar spine lengthening with body displacement, and body shortening with some trunk twisting; lower extremity braces and pedalling; upper extremity hand dabs directed to and contacting head, face, knees and uterine wall. Notable segments included two long duration sequences of rhythmic trunk extension of moderate force quality (shown as "a" in diagram).

Impression: Apparently normal movement in 14-week fetus. Diagram depicts a sample of the regulated flow of movement characteristic of this fetus at this time.

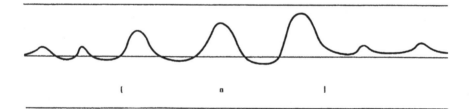

ducted using a 10-second intermittent signal with each scorable segment of tape being subjected to an alternating 10-second observation, followed by a 10-second scoring. Consensus on observations using this approach was achieved by two examiners scoring all the tapes. Based on this evaluation, the category of BMF was modified and numbers were assigned to its items for ease in data entry.

Results of Phase 3 were presented for feedback to local (Division of Physical Therapy, University of North Carolina at Chapel Hill, Research Colloquium, May, 1989), regional (Sheltering Arms Rehabilitation Hospital, Richmond, VA, June, 1989; Children's Hospital, Boston, MA, August, 1989), and a national[28] physical therapy conference. Results indicated that: (1) scoring using the assessment differentiated two out of eight subjects as outliers, (2) individual dif-

FIGURE 2. Narrative "Impression" of total 30-minute imaging and "Flow Diagram" of typical movement of Subject 3 at 14 weeks of gestation (from 10:30.00 to 11:00.00 minutes).

The 30-minute tape segment contained four movement segments ranging from 2-10 minutes. There were three rest periods from < 1 minute to 2 minutes. The view was primarily of the upper two-thirds of the body, sagittal view. Cervical-thoracic extension pattern with jaw-opening appeared repeatedly, as many as 40 times in succession, varying in force quality, use of space, and duration. This pattern occasionally led to total body displacement against gravity, followed by floating to resume shaping of the body to the uterine cavity. Shaping changes were primarily lengthening and shortening. Upper extremities were observed in far reach over the head lasting > 15 seconds. Other actions included: hand-to-face, tuck, hand dab, bilateral hands-to-head, head rotation, arm glide with far reach to uterine wall, and bilateral foot brace. Large variations occurred in force quality from 1,2 (small body part moving slowly–a) to 5,4 (whole body moving moderately fast–b).

Impression: Movement of 14-week fetus under stress, unknown etiology. Diagram depicts a sample of the irregular flow of movement characteristic of this fetus.

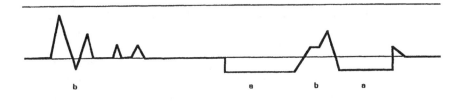

ferences in the quality of fetal movement appeared to exist, and (3) further description of specific motor behaviors was needed.

Phase 4: *Continuity with Neonatal Assessment.* Our qualitative observations, along with Milani Comparetti's and Prechtl's emphasis on continuity of fetal and neonatal movement, led us to examine the neonatal assessments of Als[29] and Brazelton[30] for identifying specific behaviors. Consultation with testers certified in use of the Neonatal Individualized Developmental Care and Assessment Program (NIDCAP), Assessment of Premature Infant Behavior (APIB)[29] and Brazelton Neonatal Behavioral Assessment Scale (BNBAS),[30] and BNBAS certification of the senior author, resulted in the incorporation into the Q-MOVE of portions of the neurobehavioral categorization of infant motor behaviors described by Als and Brazelton. Behaviors added to the scale were based on MacLeod's[31] application of the Als system to fetal movement and provided a substantial contribution to the accurate description of the behavioral repertoire of the fetus. These behaviors completed the development of the second part of the Q-MOVE, the Actions and Action Sequences.

The assessment of force continued to be problematic, so the authors consulted a physical therapist who specialized in biomechanics (Personal communication, Dr. Cheryl Riegger-Krugh, July, 1990). Through this consultation, the force quality portion of the Q-MOVE was modified, and research was begun on quantitative measurement of angular velocity for the purpose of validating our qualitative categorizations. Concurrent with this work, the senior author participated in Dr. Riegger-Krugh's course on Developmental Biomechanics, engaging in fetal dissection with emphasis on joint development. This effort documented initial joint development and full muscle form by 10 weeks.

Phase 5: Organizational Summary. Full data analysis was conducted of a random sample of three subjects' movement at 12, 14, and 18 weeks GA. Using 100 frames per second for detailed analysis, these tapes were scored for Actions and Action Sequences. The Actions and Action Sequences were then characterized according to the BMF, again using 100 frames per second. Seven additional tapes were viewed to further refine the **Q-MOVE** descriptions. No additional behaviors were identified on observation of these imagings. Review of the 18 imagings during this phase led to an initial categorization of some essential components of fetal motor coordination. This process is highly complex and will be the focus of future systematic study.

RESULTS

The Qualitative Assessment of Fetal Movement (Q-MOVE) is composed of three parts: Basic Movement Factors, Actions and Action Sequences, and an Organizational Summary (Table 2).

Basic Movement Factors

The Basic Movement Factors (BMF) of the **Q-MOVE** are the individual factors of Spatial Use, Timing and Force Quality. The components of these factors are shown in Tables 3, 4 and 5. In using the Q-MOVE, these items are given specific numbers to assist in data entry.

Spatial Use. As shown in Table 3, Spatial Use by the fetus combines three sub-factors: **Shaping** in relation to the uterine environment, **Limb Excursion, and Spatial Limb Paths**. Shaping concerns the dynamic progression of gross and fine movement that appears to help the fetus accommodate to the uterine environment. The spatial environment for the fetus consists of the uterine cavity, amniotic fluid, placenta, and umbilical cord. Within this environment, the fetus extends or lengthens, flexes or shortens, abducts or widens, adducts or narrows, and twists or rotates. Limb excursions can occur close or near to the fetus, or extend away from the fetus toward the uterine wall. The direction or paths of the movements can be direct or focused, indirect or meandering, or can occur within several planes, e.g., diagonal limb movements. Because of the two-dimensional nature of the imagings, the Effort-Shape language better describes the movement character.

Timing. Temporal patterning of fetal movements may be qualitatively differentiated in terms of **Continuity** and **Duration** as shown

Table 3. Spatial Use Subfactors of the Basic Movement Factors

SPATIAL USE

Shaping	Limb Excursion	Spatial Paths
Lengthening, shortening	Near	Direct/focal
Widening, narrowing	Intermediate	Indirect/meandering
Twists	Far	Other

Table 4. Timing Patterns of the Basic Movement Factors

TIMING

Continuity	Duration
Discrete	Brief
Sequential	Moderate
Continuous	Long
Discontinuous	

Table 5. Force Quality Parameters of the Basic Movement Factors

FORCE QUALITY

Mass

Small	Medium	Large	Extra Large
hand	lower leg	trunk	trunk & head
foot	upper limb	lower limb(s)	trunk & limb(s)
finger(s)	head		whole body

Angular Velocity

slow	moderately fast
moderately slow	fast
moderate	

in Table 4. **Continuity** refers to the way movements are sequenced. The four variations in **Continuity** are **discrete, sequential, continuous and discontinuous. Duration** of Actions is assessed in terms of **brief** (< 2 seconds), **moderate** (2-4 seconds) or **long** (> 4 seconds).

"**Discrete**" refers to individual movements with a recognizable beginning and end followed by a pause, e.g., a kick.[31] "**Sequential**" refers to a series of different Discrete Actions strung together without pause, e.g., foot brace, hip extension, roll, tuck. "**Continuous**" refers to repetitive discrete actions or patterns in which the fetus engages for variable periods (e.g., pedalling or sucking). These movements appear to have a repetitive rhythmic nature which distinguishes them from Discrete Actions. "**Discontinuous**" refers to movements separated by short rest periods (under 2 sec), e.g., hiccoughs.

The **Timing** of Actions or Action Sequences is described and scored by combining **Continuity** and **Duration**. For example, the timing of a kick might be categorized as discrete/brief. A cervical flexion followed by trunk flexion and trunk rotation might be categorized as sequential/long. The timing of a pedalling movement could be categorized as continuous/moderate, while a lengthy sequence of hiccoughs would be discontinuous/long.

Force Quality. The exact amount of force exerted during movement by fetal trunk and limbs is impossible to ascertain through two-dimensional observation. Force measurements cannot be determined at this time because standardized measures for fetal segmental masses at successive gestational ages and for amniotic fluid viscosities have not been established. We define "force quality," therefore, as a relative descriptor of the apparent degree of force applied during movement. We indicate force quality using two numbers. The first number indicates a segmental mass of small, medium, large or extra-large size. For example, "1" indicates a small mass: a finger, hand or foot. The second number indicates the apparent angular velocity at which the segmental mass is moving. The relative angular velocity of the movement is categorized as (1) slow, (2) moderately slow, (3) moderate, (4) moderately fast or (5) fast. The minimal force quality is scored with two digits: "1,1"; maximal force quality is "4, 5." The numbers for segmental mass and apparent angular velocity designate approximate categories rather than a continuum of equal intervals of absolute values. Quantitative measurement of angular velocity is being conducted at present in order to support the qualitative assessment (Personal communication, Riegger-Krugh, Blair, Sparling, March, 1992). This approach has validated the qualitative measures with two cases as described in the paper by Riegger-Krugh in this issue.

ACTIONS AND ACTION SEQUENCES

Actions and Action Sequences are the "content" portion of the **Q-MOVE**; they are movement behaviors and patterns that occur repeatedly and are characteristic of the early fetal period. The Q-MOVE system was developed from study of 18 normal subjects from 12 to 18 weeks of gestation. We assume, therefore, that the categories of the Q-MOVE are inclusive of the movements of normal subjects of this age range. All of the fetal movements observed so far can be categorized as either Actions or Action Sequences. When the system is applied to impaired or abnormal fetuses, additional movements or patterns characteristic of specific disabilities may well be identified.[32-34] As greater numbers of subjects are studied, differences may become diagnostic.

From the large number of Actions and Action Sequences (Table 6), several will be described. Actions include central body and peripheral movements. An Action Sequence is comprised of several Actions strung together in combination without long pauses, e.g., leg brace-roll-tuck, and could be characterized for "timing" as a sequential action of long duration. **Actions of the Central Body** include 14 behaviors such as the "arch/stretch" which is defined as "extension of cervical and thoracic spine; may be accompanied by bilateral, unilateral arm extension or leg extension; similar to retroflexion of the head described by deVries et al.[2]" The "tuck," referred to by Als[29] as "trunkal tucking," occurs with flexion of the trunk, head, spine and lower extremities.

Actions of the Peripheral Body include three arm, nine hand, six leg, four foot, and five head/neck movements. The "arm glide" refers to "smooth and continuous arm excursion covering multiple spatial points, relatively low force quality." The "hand clasp" is a common behavior noted by Als[29] in observing the premature infant. Hands are "positioned against one another, usually in midline." The "leg brace" describes the movement of "legs extended, feet touching uterine wall or other support point." The "foot clasp" is another behavior noted by Als[29] in the premature infant describing "feet positioned against one another." "Head brace" describes "the head pressed against the uterine wall with the posture sustained for some period." Action Sequences can consist of a combination of any number of central and peripheral body actions. "Build up" is "a repeated trunk flexion or extension which appears to increase in tempo over a 2-10 second period."

SUMMARY ORGANIZATION

The third section of the Q-MOVE, outlined in Table 2, is a summary impression of the health status of the fetus as evidenced by its observed motor behavior. The summary is presented in narrative format. A 30-second flow chart of a small but typical sample of the subject's movement is also presented.

Narrative Format. Based on our observations to date with normal subjects, the following aspects of fetal movement are thought to be significant indicators of the normally maturing fetus. Descrip-

Table 6. Discrete Actions and Action Sequences

DISCRETE ACTIONS

Central Body Actions   **Peripheral Actions**

	ARM	**HAND**
Arch/stretch	Glide	Dab
Displacement	Jerk	Clasp
Float	Reach	Finger splay
Jerk		Glide
Hiccough		Grasp
Push-off		Hand to head
Rib cage movement		Hand to mouth
Roll-log, segmental		Isolated
Sink		Midline
Squirm		
Stretch		
Twist	**LEG**	**FOOT**
Tuck		
Uncurl	Brace	Clasp
	Clasp	Dab
	Kick	Heel brace
	Pedalling	Toe wiggle
	Stretch	
	Thrust	

HEAD AND NECK

Anteflexion
Brace
Retroflexion
Rotation
Thrust

ACTION SEQUENCES

Build up
Hand to body part - contact-release
Hand to mouth-insert-suck-remove
Hand across midline
Pedalling
Repeated kicking - same leg
Thrust-brace-roll

tions of these characteristics form the basis of the "Impression" narrative.

1. Presence of Actions and Action Sequences
2. Variation in Action Sequence combinations
3. Repetition of Actions and Action Sequences

4. Variations in Spatial Use, Force Quality and Timing
5. Refinement of Actions and Action Sequences, i.e., hand to mouth
6. Presence of inactivity/activity cycles
7. Presence of apparently functional movements, i.e., pedalling

Prior to its clinical use, this portion of the assessment will be elaborated upon to include results of further data analysis with the Actions and Action Sequences and their qualifiers, the Basic Movement Factors.

Pictorial Format. The narrative description is a general statement of the observer's "impression" of the movement of the total imaging. A flow diagram, as shown in Figures 1 and 2, accompanies the narrative impression. These diagrams are 30-second samples of the motor activity of two fetuses during a thirty-minute imaging. They provide a means of quickly communicating the individual differences in timing and force quality of a segment of movement.

CONCLUSION

Fetal motor behavior manifests itself as a dynamic process. The fetus moves and grows within a unique context. To assess the fetus moving within its natural environment, we have developed a qualitative assessment of its movement, the Q-MOVE. Through use of this tool, investigators can be guided in observation of fetal movements that are ordered in space and time, and exhibit variations in force quality. These basic movement characteristics combine to form a variety of movement patterns, some of which, such as pedalling and reaching, may be functional. Although we do not yet understand the mechanisms of the development of fetal neuromuscular coordination,[35] this complex process is at least partly revealed in the observation of real-time fetal movement behaviors.

The future of fetal movement research with the Q-MOVE depends in part upon its application to clinical studies, such as research with fetuses of diabetic mothers. Forthcoming technological advances in ultrasound imaging will facilitate the achievement of adequate reliability and validity, paving the way for the Q-MOVE to be used for investigations of neurobehavioral development. The initial measurement of fetal movement focused on the description of reflex-based motor patterns[10,11] and later on the establishment of categories or milestones[1, 2] to describe the appearance and development of spontaneous fetal motor behaviors. Presently, motor control concepts suggest the need to study the way in which fetal motor patterns are formed, practiced and constrained in order to delineate the development of functional forms of movement.[36] The potential significance of the Q-MOVE rests with researchers who might use the tool to chart the course of prenatal motor development, differentiate low-risk from high-risk fetuses, compare qualitative aspects of prenatal and postnatal human movement, and compare fetal with maternal activities.

REFERENCES

1. Milani Comparetti A. Pattern analysis of normal and abnormal development: the fetus, the newborn, the child. In: Slaton DS, ed. Development of Movement in Infancy. Chapel Hill, NC: University of North Carolina; 1981:1-37.

2. deVries JIP, Visser GHA, Prechtl HFR. The emergence of fetal behaviour. I Qualitative aspects. *Early Hum Dev.* 1982;7:301-322.

3. Prechtl HFR. Qualitative changes of spontaneous movements in fetus and preterm infant are a marker of neurological dysfunction. *Early Hum Dev.* 1990; 23:151-158.

4. Touwen BCL. Motility in the fetus and young infant: Implications for neurological development. *Eur J Clin Nutri.* 1989;43:27-32.

5. Bekedam DJ, Visser GHA. Effects of "hypoxemic events" on breathing, body movements, and heart rate variations: a study in growth retarded human fetuses. *Am J Obstet Gynecol.* 1985;153:52-56.

6. Mantel R, van Geijn HP, Ververs IAP, Copray FJA. Automated analysis of near-term antepartum fetal heart rate in relation to fetal behavioral states: The Sonicaid System 8000. *Am J Obstet Gynecol.* 1991;165:57-65.

7. Ehrstrom G: Circadian rhythm of fetal movements. *Acta Obstet Gynecol Scand.* 1984;63:539-541.

8. O'Dowd MJ: Quickening–a re-evaluation. *Br J Obstet Gynecol.* 1985;92: 1037-1039.

9. Prechtl, HFR. Continuity and change in early neural development. In: Prechtl H, ed.: *Continuity of Neural Functions from Prenatal to Postnatal Life.* Clinics in Developmental Medicine No. 94. Philadelphia, PA: JB LIppincott; 1984: 1-15.

10. Hooker D. *The Prenatal Origin of Behavior, 18th Porter Lecture.* Lawrence, KS: University of Kansas Press; 1952.

11. Humphrey T. Some correlations between the appearance of human fetal reflexes and the development of the nervous system. *Prog Brain Res.* 1964;4:9-133.

12. Birnholz JC, Stephens JC, Faria M. Fetal movement patterns: a possible means of defining neurologic developmental milestones in utero. *Am J Roentgenol.* 1978;130:537-540.

13. Reinold E. Ultrasonics in early pregnancy: diagnostic scanning and fetal motor activity. *Contrib Gynecol Obstet.* 1979; 1:116-127.

14. Ianniruberto A, Tajani E. Ultrasonographic study of fetal movements. *Semin Perinatol.* 1981;5(2):175-181.

15. Milani Comparetti A. The neurophysiologic and clinical implications of studies on fetal motor behavior. *Sem Perinatol.* 1981;5(2):183-189.

16. McGuiness-Scott J. Movement Study and Benesh Movement Notation. London: Oxford University Press; 1983:1-23.

17. Cohen LR: Labanalysis for the social scientist with a general systems perspective. Dance Research Annual IX, Congress on Research in Dance. New York, NY: New York University; 1978:145-154.

18. Bartenieff I, Lewis D. Body Movement. New York, NY: Gordon and Breach Science Publishers; 1980:viii-ix.

19. Kestenberg J. The role of movement patterns in development. *Psychoanal Q.* 1965;34:1-36, 517-563.

20. Kestenberg J, Sossin M. The Role of Movement Patterns in Development. New York, NY: New York Dance Notation Bureau Press; 1979:153-154.

21. Eshkohl N, Wachmann A. *Movement Notation.* London: Weidenfeld and Nicholson; 1958.

22. Golani I, Fentress J. Early ontogeny of face grooming in mice. *Dev Psychobiol.* 1985;18(6):529-544.

23. Fentress JC. Developmental roots of behavioral order: systematic approaches to the examination of core developmental issues. In: Gunnar MR, Thelen E, eds. *Systems and Development. The Minnesota Symposia on Child Psychology*, Volume 22. Hillsdale, NJ: Lawrence Erlbaum; 1989:47-51.

24. Benesh R, Benesh J. *An Introduction to Benesh Dance Notation.* London: A & C Black; 1956.

25. Milani Comparetti A, Gidoni EA. A graphic method of recording normal and abnormal movement patterns. *Dev Med Child Neurol.* 1968;10:633-636.

26. Szostek TK. *Observational Coding System.* Research Triangle Park, NC: Research Triangle Collaborative; 1988.

27. Green S. Application of effort-shape theory to fetal movement study. *Pediatric Physical Therapy.* 1989;1(1):20.

28. Sparling JW, Wilhelm IJ. Qualitative assessment of fetal arm movements. *Phys Ther.* 1989;69:397.

29. Als H. Manual for the Naturalistic Observation of Newborn Behavior (Preterm and Fullterm Infants). Boston, MA: The Children's Hospital; 1984.

30. Brazelton TB. Neonatal Behavioral Assessment Scale, 2nd Edition. Clinics in Developmental Medicine 88. Philadelphia, PA: JB Lippincott; 1984.

31. MacLeod AM. The development of fetal behaviors and their relationship to neonatal behavioral organization. Unpublished Master of Science thesis. Chapel Hill, NC: University of North Carolina at Chapel Hill; 1990.

32. Visser GHA, Laurini RN, deVries JIP, Bekedam DJ, Prechtl HFR. Abnormal motor behavior in anencephalic fetuses. *Early Hum Dev.* 1985;12:173-182.

33. Visser GHA, Bekedam DJ, Mulder EJH, Ballegooie E van. Delayed emergence of fetal behavior in type-I diabetic women. *Early Hum Dev.* 1985; 12:167-172.

34. Bekedam DJ, Visser GHA, deVries JJ, Prechtl HFR. Motor behavior in the growth retarded fetus. *Early Hum Dev.* 1985;12:155-165.

35. Fentress JC. The development of coordination. *J Motor Behav.* 1984;16(2): 99-134.

36. Schmidt RA. *Motor Control and Learning: A Behavioral Emphasis*, second edition. Champaign, IL: Human Kinetics Publishers; 1988.

Behavioral States
in the Human Fetus

Irma J. Wilhelm

SUMMARY. The development of behavioral states is described in the full-term and premature neonate and in the human fetus. Various methods of classifying behavioral states are reviewed and contrasted. Clinical implications of fetal state assessment are prsented in terms of the practice of obstetrics and the prediction of neonatal neurologic outcome.

Behavioral states of sleeping and waking, sometimes termed states of consciousness, have been recognized, studied, and described for a number of decades in humans and animals of all ages.[1-5] Animals of many species exhibit very similar state-related behavior through patterns of overt activity and physiologic reactions.[5] The behavioral state of an organism affects all other behavior and, therefore, must be either measured or controlled during any behavioral observation or assessment.[5,6]

A behavioral state consists of a cluster of clearly defined behavioral and physiologic variables that occur together, are stable in time and tend to recur.[7-10] One of these variables is movement; therefore, the study of human fetal movement is intimately related to and dependent on the ability to recognize and describe behavioral states in the human fetus.

Irma J. Wilhelm, MS, PT, was Research Associate Professor in the Division of Physical Therapy, Department of Medical Allied Health Professions, School of Medicine, University of North Carolina at Chapel Hill when this paper was written. Her work was supported in part by Maternal and Child Health Postgraduate Training Grant 149, US Department of Health and Human Services.

Address for reprints: RFD 7, Box 960, Augusta, ME 04330.

The purpose of this paper is to trace the development of this ability to describe human fetal state. In order to understand the continuity of the behavioral state research, we will begin with the earliest studies, those of neonatal states, then back up gestationally and examine work related to behavioral states in the premature infant. Finally, we will regress to the (study of) fetal state. Within each topic, however, we will go forward in the sense of examining the research as it developed in time. We will conclude by examining the possible clinical implications of assessing fetal state by reviewing studies of behavioral state in high-risk and compromised fetuses.

BEHAVIORAL STATES IN THE HUMAN NEONATE

In her early work with neonates, summarized in 1977, Saint-Anne Dargassies[11] described a neurological screening method in which just one item assesses state. That item is termed "vigilance" and is defined as ". . . a quality of alertness such that the infant exhibits both receptivity and reactivity."[11,p144] The vigilant infant is further described as able to accept or refuse to respond to a stimulus, and as being able to stay awake without crying as if in expectation. She considered impairment of vigilance to be a serious symptom in newborn infants considered "suspect" or "pathological."

A number of more complete systems for defining and classifying the behavioral states of the human neonate have been developed. The various authors of the systems do not always concur on exactly what properties should be used to distinguish one state from another, nor on how many states can be defined, nor on how long a collection of properties must last before a state can be declared present. Some of these differences stem from differing underlying conceptualizations of state, some from the differing backgrounds of the proponents, and some from the differing purposes for which the state classification systems were developed.[5,12] The state categories included in each classification system are shown in Table 1, and examples of how some variables are described in each system appear in Table 2.

Table 1.--Neonatal Behavioral State Classification Systems

States	Wolff	Prechtl	Brazelton	Thoman Primary	Thoman Summary
Number	7	5	6	10	6
Sleep States	Regular Sleep	State 1	State 1 Deep Sleep	Quiet Sleep	Quiet, Sleep& Active-quiet Transition sleep
	Irregular Sleep	State 2	State 2 Light sleep	Active Sleep	Active Sleep
	Periodic Sleep	-----	-----	Active-quiet Transition Sleep	
Transition States	Drowsiness	-----	State 3 Drowsy	Drowse	Drowse,Daze& Sleep-wake Transition
				Daze	
				Sleep-wake Transition	
Awake States	Alert In-activity	State 3	State 4 Alert	Alert	Alert
	Waking Activity	State 4	State 5 Eyes open, active	Nonalert Waking	Non-alert Waking
	-----	-----	-----	Fuss	-----
	Crying	State 5	State 6, Crying	Cry	Fuss and Cry

Table 2.--Sample Descriptions of Neonatal Behavioral State Parameters

Description	Wolff	Prechtl	Brazelton	Thoman
Respirations in Quiet Sleep State	Even, regular rhythm, constant amplitude	Regular	Regular breathing	Relatively slow, regular and abdominal in nature
Eyes in Quiet Awake State	Open and have a "bright, shining" appearance	Open	Open with bright look	Open, bright and shining, attentive, scanning
Motor Activity in Crying	Vigorous diffuse motor activity	Gross movements	High motor activity	

Wolff[1] was the first individual to suggest an all-inclusive state classification system (Table 1). From naturalistic observations of the spontaneous behavior of newborn infants, he described seven states and examined the threshold to external and internal stimulation in the various states. He held that states could be usefully described either as a quantitative continuum of arousal or as stable substructures of the whole organism identified by selected, discontinuous, descriptive categories. The major variables used to distinguish states were motor activity, respiration, and eye movements (Table 2). For some states, skin color and vocalizations were also described.

Prechtl[3] considers states as reflecting distinct neural mechanisms, and avoids using descriptive names and interpretations for state categories (Table 1). He prefers to describe states by five simple, mutually exclusive, numbered categories, using the dichotomized variables of eyes open or closed, respiration irregular or regular, movements present or absent, and vocalization present or absent (Table 2). Although these are the primary variables, he also describes other variables or "concomitants" which sometimes, but not invariably, occur in differing patterns dependent on state. Examples of concomitants include distinctive heart rate, electroencephalographic (EEG), and eye movement patterns. Prechtl[3] emphasizes the importance of controlling behavioral state during the neurological examination of neonates by such means as conducting the examination midway between two feeds, sequencing the test items to give the maximum probability of the infant being in the correct state, keeping manipulation of the infant to a minimum, and recording state at various points in the examination for later analysis.

Brazelton[14] uses a behaviorally-oriented state scale similar to that of Wolff[1] that includes some dichotomous and some more qualitative descriptions of six behavioral states (Tables 1 and 2). In testing infants he emphasizes the importance of interpreting infants' reactions to stimuli in relation to the infant's state, the manipulation of state by the examiner in order to obtain the best performance of the infant, and observation of the infant's "use" of state, as well as other behaviors, to control the amount of input from the environment and to signal needs to the examiner. Brazelton suggests that the pattern of states and the ability to move from one state to another may be predictors of the infant's later status.

As does Brazelton, Thoman[5] views states as a means for controlling stimulus input and for communication. She conceptualizes state organization within General Systems Theory, arguing that state as a behavioral system has the characteristics associated with system dynamics: feedback is ongoing within the system, equilibrium is maintained by the system, and constant interaction occurs among the complex variables of the system. She deliberately has named the states and described them with specific qualitative statements that are quite continuous in nature (Tables 1 and 2). She has also attempted to describe a complete taxonomy of infant behavioral states, expanding upon Wolff's original state categories. The taxonomy includes 10 Primary States, sometimes collapsed into 6 Summary States, that are highly interrelated. She also includes additional properties such as skin color, muscle tone, and facial movements or expressions in the state descriptions.

Most investigators agree that neonates demonstrate two sleep states and describe them with some consistency as having differing parameters of body, eye, and respiratory activity. Most also agree on the waking states–two or three with eyes open and differing levels of motor activity or fussy vocalizations, and one involving the intense vocalizations of crying.

The primary differences in the scales lie with the issues of transitions between and within state categories. Wolff, Thoman and Brazelton[1,5,14] recognize one or more transitional states between sleep and waking, while Prechtl[3] considers drowsiness a transition, but not a separate state. Thoman[5] differentiates three transitional states between sleep and waking (drowse, daze, sleep-wake transition) that have differing parameters of eye opening, motor activity and vocalizations. She also recognizes a transitional state between active and quiet sleep which may correspond to the state that Wolff[1] described as periodic sleep (Table 1).

The amount of time that state parameters must be simultaneously present in order to be called an actual state varies rather widely among investigators and, most likely, contributes to some of the disagreement about transitions. Prechtl[3] only recognizes changes lasting three minutes or more as representing new states; Brazelton[14] counts 15 second changes; while Thoman[5] records any recognizable change as a state change, regardless of how long it lasts. Thus, Brazelton and Thoman do, and Prechtl does not, recognize short-lasting transitions as states.

The fact that behavioral states are so well developed in the full-term healthy neonate, has led to a number of questions such as: can behavioral states be identified in the premature neonate, can states be recognized at any gestational age, and do premature infant states differ from those of full-term infants?

BEHAVIORAL STATES IN THE PRETERM HUMAN NEONATE

Most investigators[3,5] use the same behavioral state classification systems developed for full-term neonates for identifying premature infant states. Thoman states: "We have found this classification of states, termed Primary States to be appropriate for premature and full-term infants, and we have found them to be applicable throughout the first year of life, with no indication that they should not continue to apply at older ages."[5,p97] Prechtl and colleagues[15] reported that the state variables of respiration, activity and eye movements are independent of each other, although they may occasionally overlap by chance, until the premature infant reaches about 36 weeks postconceptional age (PCA).

In contrast, Als and associates, although not claiming that premature infants have stable behavioral states, have observed that ". . . it is possible to make meaningful systematic distinctions between dynamic transformations of various behavioral configurations which appear to correspond to varying states of availability and conscious responsiveness."[16,p74] The behavioral configurations observed during administration of the Assessment of Premature Infant Behavior (APIB) are eye movements, eye opening, facial expressions, body movements, respiration, and muscle tone. Two levels of states are classified: "A" states are described as noisy, unclean, diffuse (premature infant states); "B" states are described as clean and well-defined (full-term infant states). Six states, corresponding to those of Brazelton[14] are defined within each level. In addition the notation of "AA" is used to denote states of extreme disorganization in which the infant becomes diffusely unreachable (e.g., with severe apnea, bradycardia, cyanosis, gastro-intestinal upset, total flaccidity). States are assigned as soon as they are recognizable (e.g., lasting about 3 seconds or more).

Curzi-Dascalova et al.[17] determined that active and quiet sleep can be distinguished in the preterm infant as early as 31 weeks using the concordance of EEG and rapid eye movements (REMs) as criteria. In premature infants at all ages, other criteria (e.g., respiration, electromyography, body movements) had poor concordance which could explain the lack of consensus in the literature as to the age at which sleep states first appear.

Regardless of what state classification system is used, and whether states are considered to be fully or just partially developed, most investigators agree that the most immature premature infants (e.g., 30 weeks gestation or less) spend a major portion of their time in a rather active, diffuse, poorly defined sleep state, sometimes called indeterminate, or transitional sleep.[17-19] During the premature period the sleep states become better defined and more comparable to those of the full-term neonate and waking states begin to appear. The general sequence appears to be a gradual decrease in active (REM) sleep with an increase in quiet sleep, active awake and crying, and finally quiet awake states.[17,19,20,21] Holditch-Davis[18] reported very similar state developmental patterns even in high-risk premature infants.

Comparisons of full-term and preterm infants at equivalent gestational ages generally indicate that preterm infants have longer bouts of quiet sleep, more body movement during sleep, more frequent REM episodes, more frequent state changes, and lower correspondence among sleep state criteria. Preterm infants also spend more time during the day in awake states, (perhaps because of earlier diurnal patterning).[4,18]

With the advent of methods to visualize the human fetus, the next questions to be addressed were: can behavioral states or their precursors be identified in the fetus, what form do they take and what parameters can be used to classify them?

BEHAVIORAL STATES
IN THE NEAR-TERM HUMAN FETUS

Early Studies Using External Monitoring Techniques

Before the technology of ultrasonography was available for visualization of the human fetus, investigators attempted to study fetal behavioral states using various external monitoring techniques such as cardiotocography and tocodynamometry. Using these external techniques, Timor-Tritsch et al.[22] classified behavioral states in fetuses between 38 and 40 weeks of gestation. One-minute epochs were termed "active," "quiet," or "intermediate/transitional" depending on measurements of fetal movement and fetal heart rate (FHR) long-term variability and baseline rates. The authors documented the percent of observed time spent in and the average durations of each of these states. In another study Timor-Tritsch et al.[23] described fetal respiratory patterns in relation to fetal states. They detected regular respiratory patterns only during the quiet periods and irregular respiratory patterns in active and intermediate periods. They speculated that fetal quiet periods are probably analogs of neonatal non-REM (NREM) sleep. Fetal active periods could not be discriminated, as they might represent either REM sleep or waking, active states.

In a series of studies, Junge[24-26] also attempted to classify near-term and post-term fetal states through external monitoring of FHR and motor activity patterns. He classified the states as assumed NREM and REM sleep and wakefulness based on the similarities to neonatal state parameters, and described total times, mean durations of, and percents of observation time spent in these assumed states. He also described the ratios of assumed NREM to REM sleep states and FHR and motor activity patterns in assumed NREM and REM states, and compared these parameters in the near-term and post-term fetus and the neonate. He concluded that the similarities between fetal and neonatal parameters strongly suggest that ". . . in the fetus as in the newborn a regular change of central nervous coordination does exist and the spontaneously changing central nervous coordination or arousal is the predominating factor governing antepartum FHR pattern and its variation in fetal wellbeing."[25,p145]

Martin and Nijhuis et al.[8, 10] enumerated the problems inherent in these early observations, namely that both FHR and its variability are affected by fetal activity. The observed "states" defined only by those parameters, therefore, could be simply cycles of fetal activity and nonactivity. In addition, fetal breathing cannot be used as a state variable because the fetus does not breathe all the time. Essentially, then, the early investigators were defining state with only one variable–fetal motility.

Studies Using Ultrasonography

In order for true states to be delineated, at least two variables, preferably more, must simultaneously meet clearly defined criteria, must recur in the same combinations, must change parameters nearly simultaneously, and must last a minimum duration of time. State variables used for neonates (respiratory patterns, eyelid opening and closing, EEG patterns) cannot be used to determine the existence of fetal states. With the combination of real-time ultrasonography and FHR monitoring, at least three variables can be observed as measures of fetal states: fetal motility, rapid or slow eye movements, and heart rate patterns.[8-10,27]

Fetal states were first described by Nijhuis et al.[9,10,27] using these three parameters in near term (38-40 week) fetuses. Body movements were monitored with one real-time ultrasound transducer and eye movements were observed with a second transducer with signals stored on videotape. The body movements were verbally described and recorded on the voice channel of the videotape. The FHR was monitored with conventional cardiotocography synchronized with the videotape using an event marker. Recording sessions lasted 1-2 hours. The FHR and motility records were aligned and the resulting graphic display was analyzed with a three-minute moving window technique for those patterns of FHR, eye movements and body movements that met the criteria of stability, simultaneity of change and recurrence required for delineation of a behavioral state.

Four fetal states were recognized which resembled the neonatal states 1, 2, 3, and 4 described by Prechtl[3] and were designated states 1F to 4F:[8-10, 27]

1F: Body movements–absent except for brief gross movements, mostly startles

Eye movements–absent

Heart rate pattern A (FHRP-A)–stable, small oscillation bandwidth (usually less than 10 bpm), only isolated accelerations strictly related to movements

2F: Body movements–frequent gross and smaller movements (stretching and retroflexion of trunk; movements of extremities, head and face)

Eye movement–present (REMs and SEMs) continually

Heart rate pattern B (FHRP-B)–wider oscillation bandwidth than A (10-15 bpm); frequent accelerations during movements (10-20 bpm)

3F: Body movements–absent

Eye movements–present continually

Heart rate pattern C (FHRP-C)–stable, wider oscillation bandwidth than A, no accelerations

4F: Body movements–frequent, continual, vigorous activity including trunk rotations

Eye movements–present continually

Heart rate pattern D (FHRP-D)–unstable, with large and long-lasting accelerations (25-30 bpm), frequently fused into a sustained tachycardia

Using this system Nijhuis et al.[9, 10] studied the fetuses of multigravidae with uncomplicated, singleton pregnancies which all resulted in deliveries of healthy, full-term infants. They reported that true states could be identified in a few fetuses at 36 weeks gestation, and in all fetuses at 38 and 40 weeks. Before those ages, the periods of coincidence of parameters of the state variables were short and periods of discordance relatively long. The requirement of simultaneity of change within three minutes was not satisfied in most fetuses until 38 weeks. van Vliet et al.[28] using the same methodology, reported that, in general, the fetuses of nulliparous women demonstrated the same patterns of state development as seen in the multiparae. The one exception was that the fetuses of the nulliparae developed true states somewhat later in gestation than those of the multiparae (e.g., no nulliparous fetus had states at 36 weeks, and one had no states by 40 weeks). In a more recent study, van Woerden et al.[29] reported significantly more time spent in state 1F by fetuses of multiparous women, than by those of nulliparae.

A number of other variables have been found to be state-related but, because they are not continuously present in the fetal period, cannot be used as state criteria. Still, if present, they can be helpful in identifying fetal states. These are fetal breathing movements, micturition, and mouthing movements.[9,10,27,30-33] Fetal breathing movements are more regular during state 1F than 2F and have a higher incidence in 2F than 1F. They appear to be irregular during 4F, but recording is not reliable because of the high general activity level in this state. Fetal voiding appears to be inhibited during state 1F, but occurs frequently during or after a change to state 2F. Regular mouthing movements (repeated small movement clusters of mouth or chin) also appear to be a concomitant of state 1F, while jaw opening, tongue protrusion, yawning and grimacing are more typical of state 2F. The characteristics of regular mouthing movements in the fetus are very similar to those of non-nutritive sucking in the neonate. van Woerden et al.[32] have identified differing heart rate patterns within state 1F that are dependent on the presence or absence of fetal breathing and mouth movements. They question, therefore, whether FHR should be considered a state concomitant rather than a state variable (as it is for the neonate).

The near-term fetus spends the majority of its time in state 2F (50-60%) and about half as much in state 1F (25-30%). States 3F and 4F are much less frequently observed, and no state can be identified about 5-10% of the time.[8-10,29,34]

Although true states meeting all requirements of stability and simultaneity of change do not appear to occur in fetuses less than 36 weeks of postconceptional age, studies of the occurrence of state precursors at younger ages have provided some information on how states develop. The studies to be reviewed are those in which two or more state-related variables were included, as opposed to studies in which only fetal movement or fetal rest and activity cycles were examined.

EARLY FETAL STATE DEVELOPMENT

Arduini et al.[35] studied the development of fetal active, quiet and transitory phases and other state-related variables longitudinally in healthy fetuses at two-week intervals from 28 weeks gestation to term. They reported that at 28-32 weeks, percent durations of active and transitory phases were significantly higher and quiet phases significantly lower than at 38-42 weeks.

The study of Nijhuis et al.[9,10] involved longitudinal examination of the fetuses of multigravidae from 32 to 40 weeks. They reported developmental trends for each state-related variable, as well as the developmental course of the coincidence of state 1F and 2F variable parameters. The separate developmental trends of the variables showed extreme individual variability and shed very little light on the development of fetal states. The only developmental trends that could be summarized for all fetuses were increases in the mean durations of FHRP A, and absent eye and body movements with increasing maturity, especially between 36 and 38 weeks of gestation.

The term "coincidence of state parameters" was used to describe periods of time in which fetuses displayed all three state parameters that describe a fetal state, but did not satisfy the other criteria for declaration of a state, namely duration or simultaneity of change. For state 1F, coincidence of parameters occurred as early as 32 weeks, but the median duration was only 6.5 minutes. A major increase in median duration of state 1F occurred only at 38 weeks when it was 22.5 minutes. Through 36 weeks, therefore, the parameters are largely independent and may appear together only by chance.

For state 2F no major change in median duration of parameter coincidence was evident; the median duration at 32 weeks was 8 minutes and at 40 weeks had risen to only 11 minutes. States 3F and 4F did not show a developmental course. State 3F occurred too infrequently to be measured, while state 4F was characterized by so much motor activity that eye movements could not always be observed reliably. In addition, FHRP D was so closely linked to state 4F motor activity that these parameters virtually never occurred separately, thus obscuring the study of the development of coincidence. The authors concluded that fetal state development closely paralleled state development in the low-risk preterm infant, as described by Prechtl et al.,[15] and that episodes of state parameter coincidence occurring before 36-38 weeks should not be considered states. In addition, fetuses of nulliparae did not differ from those of multiparae in development of state parameter coincidence.[28]

Visser et al.[36] examined fetal behavioral state variables in healthy nulliparous women at 30-32 weeks of gestation. They reported the relationship between FHRP A and FHRP B, C, and D combined (and termed B) and low vs. high incidence of fetal body and eye movements. The results indicated that during FHRP A both eye and body movements were of low incidence 57% of the observation time; while during FHRP B they were high 74% of the time. The authors also examined the changes in eye and body movements following a change in FHR pattern. The eye and body movements changed in the appropriate direction within six minutes in 71% of the FHR changes and within four minutes in 48%, and in no case did the movements change in an inappropriate direction within six minutes. These percentages differed significantly from those expected, if the pattern changes of the three variables were totally independent of each other. The investigators concluded that ". . . at 30 to 32 wk of gestation heart rate variation and eye and gross body movements are not independent variables and that coordination among the cyclic patterns of these variables is present well before 36 wk."[36, p658]

In a recent study, Swartjes et al.[37] examined the clustering of fetal movements at 20 weeks, and the coincidence of fetal state parameters at 32 and 38 weeks gestation in women with uneventful singleton pregnancies that resulted in the delivery of neurologically normal neonates. At 20 weeks, 17 periods of absent body movements lasting more than 3 minutes were recorded, a figure significantly higher than the single such period expected by chance. At 32 weeks, the percent of the recording time in which coincidences of states 1F through 4F were recorded was 59%, compared with 22.6% expected by chance, but no fetuses had true behavioral states. At 38 weeks more coincidence was found than at 32 weeks, the amount also differing significantly from that expected by chance (80% versus 30%), and 50% of the fetuses had true fetal states. The authors, therefore, concur with the results of Visser et al.[36] that state parameters at 30-32 weeks are clearly coordinated. The results of the latter two studies suggest a gradual development of states as opposed to a sudden emergence of fully coordinated states at 36-38 weeks.

Arduini et al.[38] conducted a longitudinal study of the development of transitions between states 1F and 2F in healthy fetuses from 28 weeks until birth. Their data showed a significant decrease in duration of transitions with increasing maturity. They also noted that the sequence of change in the behavioral state variables was random until 30 weeks for 1F to 2F transitions and until 34 weeks for 2F to 1F transitions. After those ages, FHR became the first variable to change during 1F to 2F transitions and fetal body movements were first to change for 2F to 1F transitions.

If the fetus does indeed have definable behavioral states, or at least the analogs of neonatal states, is this of any importance clinically? Assessment of fetal state would appear to be important in several general areas: (1) in obstetrical assessment because of the state-dependency of the variables (FHR, fetal movement) used to assess fetal well-being and (2) in assessing the integrity of the nervous system in attempts to predict neonatal outcome.

CLINICAL IMPLICATIONS OF FETAL STATE ASSESSMENT

Obstetrical Assessment

In obstetrical assessment of fetal well-being, the reduced FHR variability and absence of FHR accelerations and fetal movement of a normal fetus in a quiet state (1F) must be distinguished from those factors observed in a compromised, depressed fetus. Since periods of quiet sleep can last as long as 30-75 minutes, extension of non-stress monitoring time perhaps to a full hour may be needed to make this differentiation.[8, 22, 24, 26, 27, 34] Pillai and James[39] suggest that, in late pregnancy, the absence of regular fetal mouthing movements may be a better indication of fetal compromise than other variables because they occur more frequently than do fetal breathing and body movements in the near term fetus. Similarly, bursts of fetal sucking may produce a sinusoidal-like FHR pattern similar to the pattern considered indicative of fetal distress. Sustained accelerations of FHR with vigorous fetal body movements may be mistaken for tachycardia with decelerations, another worrisome finding.[27]

Pillai et al.[40] described a case of severe intrauterine growth retardation with no apparent etiology in a fetus at 36 weeks gestation. Behavioral state assessment revealed no behavioral states and no cyclicity of behavior, absent mouthing movements, shallow fetal breathing, only isolated somatic movements, and FHR acceleration with every movement. The baby died one hour after Caesarian section delivery and, upon autopsy, was diagnosed with the lethal syndrome of Smith-Lemli-Opitz Type II. In this fetus the biophysical profile scores[41] were equivocal but never abnormal and the non-stress test was normal.

Prediction of Neonatal Neurologic Outcome

If the integrity of the fetal nervous system is to be examined via behavioral states for predictive purposes, the validity of fetal behavioral state assessment must be established. One step in this process would be to examine fetal state behavior in fetuses known to be in potentially compromising situations. To this end, studies have been conducted of state behavior in growth-retarded fetuses, fetuses of diabetic women, fetuses with known neurologic problems and congenital anomalies, and fetuses of mothers exposed to various drugs.

Growth Retardation. van Vliet et al.[42] studied the development of behavioral states in growth-retarded fetuses ranging in gestational age from 32 to 40 weeks (all with subsequent birthweights below the 10th percentile). They compared their data with that of Nijhuis et al.[9] and van Vliet et al.[28] obtained from low-risk multiparae and nulliparae respectively. The proportions of coincidence of state parameters did not differ in the growth-retarded fetuses at 32-38 weeks of gestational age. At 40 weeks, however, the growth-retarded fetuses had significantly higher proportions of time with no coincidence evident, primarily because of asynchronous transitions and interruptions of periods of coincidence. Coincidence 1F was frequently interrupted by episodes of general movements associated with FHR accelerations. Very few growth-retarded fetuses exhibited true states at 40 weeks compared with the low-risk groups. In addition, the movements of the growth-retarded fetuses were noted to be slow and monotonous.

Rizzo et al.[43] and Arduini et al.[44] reported similar results when comparing state transitions of near-term growth-retarded and healthy fetuses examined between 36 and 38 weeks of gestation. They noted increased incidence of periods of no coincidence of state parameters, and a decreased incidence of coincidence 1F in growth-retarded fetuses. These results were particularly evident in growth-retarded fetuses with severely increased peripheral vascular resistance as measured by pulsed Doppler ultrasonography. The growth-retarded fetuses also had longer durations of transitions between periods of coincidence than did the low-risk group, therefore, no true behavioral states were detected. In addition, growth-retarded fetuses showed the randomness of sequence in the order of change in variables during state transitions that was subsequently found to be typical of healthy fetuses at much younger gestational ages.[38]

Diabetes. Dierker et al.[45] compared active and quiet periods (assessed via external monitoring of FHR and fetal movements) in fetuses of insulin-dependent diabetic women at 28-32 and 36-40 weeks gestation to those of normal pregnancies examined at the same ages. In normal pregnancies, the number of active and quiet periods per hour was significantly lower and the duration of both active and quiet periods was significantly longer in the 36-40 week fetuses, than in the 28-32 week group. In the diabetic pregnancies, these differences were not found. Essentially the fetuses of diabetic pregnancies at 36-40 weeks of gestation resembled the normal fetuses at 28-32 weeks, suggesting delayed development of active-quiet cycles. These results support the reports of delayed maturation of other organ systems, growth, and motor development in fetuses of diabetic pregnancies.[46-49]

Mulder et al.[50] examined the development of the four fetal states in fetuses of well-controlled insulin-dependent diabetic women via real-time ultrasound scanning and FHR monitoring. The fetuses were examined longitudinally at two-week intervals between 32 and 40 weeks gestational age and results were compared with a control group of low-risk fetuses. A number of fetuses of the diabetic pregnancies exhibited a FHRP that resembled FHRP A but was more unstable. Fetuses of diabetic pregnancies also had an increased percentage of periods of no-coincidence of state parameters at all gestational ages, decreased coincidence of 3F and 4F, shorter duration of coincidence 2F, and more frequent interruption of coincidence 1F periods by body movements when compared to the control group–all indicators of poor organization of the state variables. True states could be identified in very few of the fetuses of diabetic pregnancies near term, primarily because of asynchrony of transitions.

Neurologic Conditions. Arduini et al.[51] studied the development of behavioral states in fetuses with hydrocephaly compared with healthy fetuses from 30 weeks of gestation until delivery. The groups did not differ as to incidence of FHR patterns at any age. During FHRP B, the hydrocephalic fetuses had significantly reduced numbers and duration of movements and percent of time moving. They also had similar reductions in breathing and eye movements. Hydrocephalic fetuses had significantly decreased incidence of all states and increased incidence of periods of no coincidence and these differences were particularly evident in four fetuses with very poor outcomes (all died within 6 months of birth).

Drug Exposure. van Geijn et al.[52] reported no differences in fetal heart rate patterns, coincidences of state variables, duration and incidence of states 1F and 2F, occurrence of movements, and duration of movements in state 2F when comparing fetuses exposed to maternal antiepileptic medication and control fetuses at 32 and 38 weeks of gestation.

Hume et al.[53] described state differentiation, organization and regulation in 20 fetuses of cocaine-abusing mothers and the relationship of fetal state to neonatal outcome and neonatal state behavior. Their results indicated that 65% exhibited some form of abnormal fetal state-related behaviors. Some behaviors were manifestations of acute fetal intoxication, some showed parallel withdrawal effects with their mothers, and some showed long-term effects of delay or disruption in fetal state organization. As neonates they demonstrated autonomic instability and state disorganization characterized by an "all or none" pattern of being difficult to arouse and inconsolable when aroused, and having little or no periods of quiet alertness. Fetal state organization successfully predicted the overall rating of newborn neurobehavioral status and the newborn state organization rating.

CONCLUSION

Even though, in this paper, we have progressed backward in time by discussing first the concept of behavioral state in the newborn infant, then in the premature infant, and last in the fetus, the similarities and continuities are fairly clear.

The most immature fetuses and premature infants and the compromised neonates all demonstrate poor differentiation of states characterized by high proportions of periods of no coincidence of state variable parameters and frequent interruptions of state coincidences by behaviors more typical of other states (e.g., excessive movement during fetal state coincidence 1F or premature infant state 1A).

Fetal and low-risk premature infant states develop in similar ways with increasing duration of state variable parameter coincidence and more synchronous state transitions. State transition synchrony is characterized by shorter duration transitions and more mature sequences of variable change during transitions.

If the technology for observing fetal behavior continues to develop and improve, the assessment of fetal state and its components (in particular fetal movement), may well fall within the province of the developmental therapist.[54] Aberrant fetal movement patterns may be predictive of which neonates will need immediate assessment and follow-up for potential developmental problems.

REFERENCES

1. Wolff PH. The causes, controls, and organization of behavior in the neonate. Psychol Issues. 1966;5(1):Monogr 17.

2. Sterman MB, Hoppenbrouwers T. The development of sleep-waking and rest-activity patterns from fetus to adult in man. In: Sterman MB, McGinty DJ, Adinolfi AM, eds. Brain Development and Behavior. New York, NY: Academic Press Inc; 1971:203-227.

3. Prechtl HFR. The behavioural states of the newborn infant (a review). Brain Res. 1974;76:185-212.

4. Davis DH, Thoman EB. Behavioral states of premature infants: implications for neural and behavioral development. Dev Psychobiol. 1987;20:25-38.

5. Thoman EB. Sleeping and waking states in infants: a functional perspective. Neurosci Biobehav Rev. 1990;14:93-107.

6. Korner AF. State as variable, as obstacle, and as mediator of stimulation in infant research. Merrill-Palmer Quarterly. 1972;18:77-94.

7. Prechtl HFR, Akiyama Y, Zinkin P, Grant DK. Polygraphic studies of the full-term newborn, I: technical aspects and qualitative analysis. In: MacKeith R, Bax M, eds. Studies in Infancy. Clinics in Developmental Medicine, No. 27. London, England: Spastics International Medical Publications in association with William Heinemann Medical Books Ltd; 1968:1-21.

8. Martin CB Jr. Behavioral states in the human fetus. J Reprod Med. 1981; 26:425-432.

9. Nijhuis JG, Prechtl HFR, Martin CB Jr, Bots RSGM. Are there behavioural states in the human fetus? Early Hum Dev. 1982;6:177-195.

10. Nijhuis JG, Martin CB Jr, Prechtl HFR. Behavioral states of the human fetus. In: Prechtl HFR, ed. Continuity of Neural Functions from Prenatal to Postnatal Life. Clinics in Developmental Medicine No. 94. Philadelphia, PA; JB Lippincott; 1984: 65-78.

11. Saint-Anne Dargassies S. Neurological Development in the Full-term and Premature Infant. New York, NY: Excerpta Medica; 1977.

12. Ashton R. The state variable in neonatal research: a review. Merrill-Palmer Quarterly. 1973;19:3-20.

13. Prechtl HFR. The Neurological Examination of the Full-term Newborn Infant. 2nd ed. Clinics in Developmental Medicine, No. 63. Philadelphia, PA: JB Lippincott; 1977.

14. Brazelton TB. Neonatal Behavioral Assessment Scale. 2nd ed. Clinics in Developmental Medicine, No. 88. Philadelphia, PA: JB Lippincott; 1984.

15. Prechtl HFR, Fargel JW, Weinmann HM, Bakker HH. Postures, motility and respiration of low-risk pre-term infants. Dev Med Child Neurol. 1979; 21: 3-27.

16. Als H, Lester BM, Tronick EZ, Brazelton TB. Manual for the Assessment of Preterm Infants' Behavior. In: Fitzgerald HE, Lester BM, Yogman MW, eds. Theory and Research in Behavioral Pediatrics. Vol 1. New York, NY: Plenum Press; 1982:65-132.

17. Curzi-Dascalova L, Peirano P, Morel-Kahn F. Development of sleep states in normal premature and full-term newborns. Dev Psychobiol. 1988;21:431-444.

18. Holditch-Davis D. The development of sleeping and waking states in high-risk preterm infants. Infant Behavior and Development. 1990;13:513-531.

19. Parmelee AH Jr, Wenner WH, Akiyama Y, Schultz M, Stern E. Sleep states in premature infants. Dev Med Child Neurol. 1967;9:70-77.

20. Korner AF, Brown BW Jr, Reade EP, Stevenson DK, Fernbach SA, Thom VA. State behavior of preterm infants as a function of development, individual and sex differences. Infant Behavior and Development. 1988;11:111-124.

21. Michaelis R, Parmelee AH, Stern E, Haber A. Activity states in premature and term infants. Dev Psychobiol. 1973;6:209-215.

22. Timor-Tritsch IE, Kierker LJ, Hertz RH, Deagan NC, Rosen MG. Studies of antepartum behavioral state in the human fetus at term. Am J Obstet Gynecol. 1978;132:524-528.

23. Timor-Tritsch IE, Dierker LJ, Hertz RH, Chik L, Rosen MG. Regular and irregular human fetal respiratory movement. Early Hum Dev. 1980;4:315-324.

24. Junge HD. Behavioral states and state related heart rate and motor activity patterns in the newborn infant and the fetus antepartum—a comparative study, I: technique, illustration of recordings, and general results. J Perinat Med. 1979; 7:85-107.

25. Junge HD. Behavioral states and state related heart rate and motor activity patterns in the newborn infant and the fetus ante partum—a comparative study, II: computer analysis of state related heart rate baseline and macrofluctuation patterns. J Perinat Med. 1979;7:134-146.

26. Junge HD. Behavioral states and state-related heart rate and motor activity patterns in the newborn infant and the fetus ante partum—a comparative study, III: analysis of sleep state-related motor activity patterns. Eur J Obstet Gynecol Reprod Biol. 1980;10:239-246.

27. Nijhuis JG. Behavioural states: concomitants, clinical implications and the assessment of the condition of the nervous system. Eur J Obstet Gynecol Reprod Biol. 1986;21:301-308.

28. van Vliet MAT, Martin CB Jr, Nijhuis JG, Prechtl HFR. Behavioural states in the fetuses of nulliparous women. Early Hum Dev. 1985;12:121-135.

29. van Woerden EE, van Geijn HP, Caron FJM, Swartjes JM, Mantel R, Arts NFT. Automated assignment of behavioural states in the human near term fetus. Early Hum Dev. 1989;19:137-146.

30. Nijhuis JG, Martin CB Jr, Gommers S, Bouws P, Bots RSGM, Jongsma HW. The rhymicity of fetal breathing varies with behavioural state in the human fetus. Early Hum Dev. 1983;9:1-7.

31. Arduini D, Rizzo G, Giorlandino C, et al. The fetal behavioural states: an ultrasonic study. Prenat Diagn. 1985;5:269-276.

32. van Woerden EE, van Geijn HP, Swartjes JM, Caron FJM, Brons JTJ, Arts NFT. Fetal heart rhythms during behavioural state 1F. Eur J Obstet Gynecol Reprod Biol. 1988;28:29-38.

33. van Woerden EE, van Geign HP, Caron FJM, van der Valk AW, Swartjes JM, Arts NFT. Fetal mouth movements during behavioural states 1F and 2F. Eur J Obstet Gynecol Reprod Biol. 1988;29:97-105.

34. Mantel R, van Geijn HP, Ververs IAP, Copray FJA. Automated analysis of near-term antepartum fetal heart rate in relation to fetal behavioral states: the Sonicaid System 8000. Am J Obstet Gynecol. 1991;165:57-65.

35. Arduini D, Rizzo G, Giorlandino C, Valensise H, Dell'acqua S, Romanini C. The development of fetal behavioural states: a longitudinal study. Prenat Diagn. 1986;6:117-124.

36. Visser GHA, Poelmann-Weejes G, Cohen TMN, Bekedam DJ. Fetal behavior at 30 to 32 weeks of gestation. Pediatr Res 1987;22:655-658.

37. Swartjes JM, van Geijn HP, Mantel R, van Woerden EE, Schoemaker HC. Coincidence of behavioural state parameters in the human fetus at three gestational ages. Early Hum Dev. 1990;23:75-83.

38. Arduini D, Rizzo G, Massacesi M, Romanini C, Mancuso S. Longitudinal assessment of behavioural transitions in healthy human fetuses during the third trimester of pregnancy. J Perinat Med. 1991;19:67-72.

39. Pillai M, James D. Human fetal mouthing movements: a potential biophysical variable for distinguishing state 1F from abnormal fetal behaviour; report of 4 cases. Eur J Obstet Gynecol Reprod Biol. 1990;38:151-156.

40. Pillai M, Garrett C, James D. Bizarre fetal behaviour associated with lethal congenital anomalies: a case report. Eur J Obstet Gynecol Reprod Biol. 1991; 39:215-218.

41. Manning FA, Platt LD, Sipos L. Antepartum fetal evaluation: development of a fetal biophysical profile score. Am J Obstet Gynecol. 1980;136:787-795.

42. van Vliet MAT, Martin CB Jr, Nijhuis JG, Prechtl HFR. Behavioural states in growth-retarded human fetuses. Early Hum Dev. 1985;12:183-197.

43. Rizzo G, Arduini D, Pennestri F, Romanini C, Mancuso S. Fetal behaviour in growth retardation: its relationship to fetal blood flow. Prenat Diagn. 1987; 7:229-238.

44. Arduini D, Rizzo G, Caforio L, Boccolini MR, Romanini C, Mancuso S. Behavioural state transitions in healthy and growth retarded fetuses. Early Hum Dev. 1989;19:155-165.

45. Dierker LJ, Pillay S, Sorokin Y, Rosen MG. The change in fetal activity periods in diabetic and nondiabetic pregnancies. Am J Obstet Gynecol. 1982;143: 181-185.

46. Gluck L, Kulovich MV. Lecithin/sphingomyelin ratios in amniotic fluid in normal and abnormal pregnancy. Am J Obstet Gynecol. 1973;115:539-546.

47. Sokol RJ, Hall PW. Fetal renal tubular function during late pregnancy and diabetes mellitus. Am J Obstet Gynecol. 1977;129:208-210.

48. Pedersen JF, Molsted-Pedersen L. Early fetal growth delay detected by ultrasound marks increased risk of congenital malformations in diabetic pregnancy. Br Med J. 1981;283:269-271.

49. Visser GHA, Bekedam DJ, Mulder EJH, van Ballegooie E. Delayed emergence of fetal behaviour in type-1 diabetic women. Early Hum Dev. 1985;12: 167-172.

50. Mulder EJH, Visser GHA, Bekedam DJ, Prechtl HFR. Emergence of behavioural states in fetuses of type-1-diabetic women. Early Hum Dev. 1987;15: 231-251.

51. Arduini D, Rizzo G, Caforio L, Mancuso S. Development of behavioral states in hydrocephalic fetuses. Fetal Ther. 1987;2:135-143.

52. van Geijn HP, Swartjes JM, van Woerden EE, Caron FJM, Brons JTJ, Arts NFT. Fetal behavioural states in epileptic pregnancies. Eur J Obstet Gynecol Reprod Biol. 1986;21:309-314.

53. Hume RF Jr, O'Donnell KJ, Stanger CL, Killam AP, Gingras JL. In utero cocaine exposure: observations of fetal behavioral state may predict neonatal outcome. Am J Obstet Gynecol. 1989;161:685-690.

54. Sparling JW, Wilhelm IJ, MacLeod AM, et al. Developing a taxonomy of fetal movement: the first step in a longitudinal collaborative study. Physical and Occupational Therapy in Pediatrics. 1990;10(1):43-46.

Periods of Activity and Inactivity in the 12-to 16-Week Fetus

T. Long
S. McCusker
J. Ruble
JW Sparling

SUMMARY. Active and inactive periods in four 12-to 16-week low risk human fetuses were studied. These periods are interpreted as precursors to the state parameter of fetal body movements. Adequate reliability on scoring videotapes of fetal activity and inactivity was achieved, but extensive training with explicit protocols was required. Results suggested that there was an increase in amount of fetal movement from 12 to 14 weeks, followed by a significant decrease in movement from 14 to 16 weeks. There was a significant increase in cycles per minute from 12 to 16 weeks. Early fetal movement was descriptively compared to newborn infant movement using the Brazelton Neonatal Behavioral Assessment Scale.

Behavioral states exist in the fetus by 36 weeks[1] and are characterized by the concurrence of fetal body movements, heart rate variations, and eye movements that last for specific temporal dura-

T. Long, S. McCusker and J. Ruble are affiliated with clinical sites in Burlington, NC, Minneapolis, MN and Washington, DC. JW Sparling, PhD, PT, OT, is Assistant Professor in the Division of Physical Therapy at the University of North Carolina at Chapel Hill. She is Project Director for the Maternal and Child Health Postgraduate Training Grant.

This study was supported in part by an Innovative Research Award from the Frank Porter Graham Research and Child Development Center, a Department of Medical Allied Health Professions Grant and the Maternal and Child Health Postgraduate Training Grant 149, DHHS.

This study was conducted in partial fulfillment of the requirements for a BS degree in Physical Therapy from the University of North Carolina at Chapel Hill.

tions, and have clear transition periods. From 30 weeks to 36 weeks, these three state behaviors are not independent but intermittently occur together, suggesting that this is a period of increasing organization of the nervous system.[2,3] Ardiuni[4] has described decreasing durations of transition periods and increasing coordination among state parameters starting at 28 weeks. Drogtrop et al.[5] demonstrated a link at 25 weeks between fetal body movements and fetal heart rate (FHR), and FHR and eye movements, but not between fetal eye and body movements. Prior to 25 weeks, observable periods of fetal activity do not occur concurrently with fetal heart rate and eye movement changes. Inactivity and activity periods, heart rate and eye movements prior to 25-36 weeks, therefore, have been studied as independent parameters or state precursors.

The frequency and duration of the state precursors of activity and inactivity in the 12- to 16-week human fetus has had limited investigation. This early period has been described as one of generation and expression of movement patterns,[6-8] and, therefore, a time to observe the development of human motor behavior. The purpose of this study is to describe early periods of activity and inactivity, adding to the literature on the development of movement as a precursor to one parameter of behavioral state, and as a marker for central nervous system development. The study significance lies in the potential for understanding and even predicting the functional development of the central nervous system.[9,10] The future identification of variations in early motor activity may help us identify results of antepartum asphyxia or trauma,[11,12] prepare us for difficult deliveries, and address the continuity between prenatal and postnatal motor behavior.

BACKGROUND

Parameters of Behavioral State

Numerous contemporary studies have explored the dimensions and role of behavioral state in the third trimester fetus. These studies are reviewed in detail by Wilhelm in this issue. Fundamental to most of these studies is the description of four fetal states:[13,14]

State 1F — essentially absent body and eye movements, a stable fetal heart rate (FHR) pattern.

State 2F — frequent gross and fine movements, continuous eye movements, frequent accelerations of FHR

State 3F — no body movements, continuous eye movements, stable FHR

State 4F — continuous and vigorous body movements, continuous eye movements, unstable FHR with accelerations.

The development of these states can be explored by an investigation of the parameters of eye movement, heart rate, and body movement.

Eye Movements. Eye movements can first be observed at 16 weeks.[15] Birnholz[10] has characterized these movements as single lateral deviations followed by a slower return. These slow movements become more rapid at 18-20 weeks. More complex rotary eye movements can be observed by 23 weeks and are dominant from 30-37 weeks, with repetitive deviations of eye movements dominant near term.

Fetal Heart Rate (FHR). The cardiovascular system is functional by 21 days.[16] Fetal heart rate (FHR) accelerations appear to occur at 6-7 weeks,[6] but without the stability required for state designation. Basal fetal heart rate decreases between 26 to 28 weeks and 30 to 32 weeks, while long-term fetal heart rate variability and the amplitude of fetal heart rate accelerations increase.[17] By 32 weeks, dependency of movement and heart rate variables is more consistent, and by 36 weeks a stable coincidence of fetal heart rate accelerations and eye movements is evident.

Movement. Understanding the development of movement requires knowledge of the first appearance of movements, the types and durations of movements, and the duration of periods without movement. The first observable "just discernible" fetal movements were observed between 7.5 and 8.5 weeks and were single events lasting from 0.5 to 2 seconds.[8] After 9 weeks postmenstrual age, these movements were no longer observed, but were supplanted by general movements or whole body movements without distinctive patterning or sequencing of body parts. These were slow and of limited amplitude at 8-9 weeks. By 10-12 weeks, the movements of head, trunk and limbs had become forceful and rapid enough to cause a shift in fetal position. After 12 weeks, the speed and amplitude of general movements varied, but usually lasted from 1-4 minutes. From 14-20 weeks, general movements appeared to be variable with an increase in amount from 12 to 14 weeks, and a decrease from 14 to 16 weeks.[18] A decrease in movement was noted from 20 to 36 weeks.[19]

Periods without movement lasted no longer than 13 minutes from 7-20 weeks,[20] with 24 minutes being the longest rest period at 24 weeks.[21] At 10-12 weeks, the median length of inactive periods was 6 minutes and 20 seconds and by 14 weeks inactive periods stabilized at 2 minutes.[20] These periods of quiescence do not have a diurnal variation at 13 weeks, but do at 20-22 weeks, with longer pauses between general movements and longer quiescent periods occurring in the morning.[22] Inactivity-activity cycles of behavior do not appear until 24 weeks. The presence of these cycles occurs in 80 percent of 29-week imagings.[23]

All observable movement patterns occur at least by 15 weeks. These movements have been characterized into 16 types: startles, hiccups, breathing, isolated arm, leg, head and jaw movements, sucking and swallowing, hand-to-face contact, stretches, yawns and rotation.[8] These same movements can be seen in the preterm and full term newborn infant although their fluency is limited due to the increased effect of gravity.

Movement of Impaired Fetuses

Significant differences in movement type and duration have been found among impaired fetuses. The movements may become monotonous, repetitive, and are either fast or slow.[24,25] Apparently the complexity and variability of movements is either diminished or lost in impaired fetuses. Inactivity-activity periods, as well as type and duration of movements, have been affected. Swartjes and associates[26] observed periods of inactivity greater than three minutes in significantly more fetuses of mothers exposed to antiepileptic drugs than in fetuses of mothers unexposed to these drugs. Even in the control fetuses, however, rest periods of three minutes were identified in over 33 percent of the subjects. In addition, the coincidence of FHR acceleration with fetal movement occurred by 24 weeks, suggesting a developmental progression in the coincidence of state variables. The designation of fetal states has been essential to the study of a variety of conditions including intrauterine growth retardation[27] and hydrocephalus.[28] Understanding the development of one of the state parameters and determination of its characteristics at early gestational periods may facilitate the early diagnosis of fetal risk.

From our earlier research,[18] an increase in amount of movement occurred from 12 to 14 weeks, and a decrease in amount of movement occurred from 14 to 16 weeks of gestation. We hypothesized that this would be a consistent finding with additional low-risk pregnancies because of the recognized increase and decrease in number of neuronal cells and synapses during this period of central nervous system development. To repeat these results differentiating movement at different gestational ages, even with a small sample size, would support our hypothesis and suggest the need for further study in this area.

Finally, some investigators[29] have described a developmental continuity from the fetal to neonatal period. deVries et al.[30] have described the potential for individual differences among fetuses. Consolidating these ideas, neonatal behavioral assessment was conducted as an exploratory extension of this study.

METHOD

Subjects

Maternal subjects were a convenience sample from a private obstetric practice at a tertiary-care hospital and were recruited by a clinic sign and referral from other women participating in the study. The four women had a mean age of 28.8 years, had a mean grade-level-completed of 19, and held high-level health care jobs. They volunteered to receive serial diagnostic ultrasound imaging for 25 minutes every 14 days from 12 to 16 weeks and permitted their neonates to be tested after birth using the Brazelton Neonatal Behavioral Assessment Scale (BNBAS).[31] Criteria for study inclusion were primigravida status, low risk pregnancy, and delivery at the University Hospitals. Mothers were professional women who worked throughout their pregnancy, were non-smokers and did not take any drugs or medication during pregnancy, and experienced a normal pregnancy and delivery.

The fetal subjects consisted of three males and one female (018). Two of the fetuses were premature (017 at 37 weeks, and 019 at 35 weeks) with a mean birthweight of 2606 grams. The two other fetuses (018, 020) were born at 40 weeks gestation with a mean weight of 3833 grams. All were classified as "healthy" at birth and at BNBAS testing at 42 weeks, a time selected in order to ensure the physiological stability of all newborn infants.

Instrumentation

Ultrasound images of real-time fetal movement were videotaped using an Ultramark 4, 3.5 MHz linear array machine with videorecorder. Later analysis was conducted using a high-resolution monitor and a superimposed time code of 100 frames per second. A software program, the Observational Coding System,[32] permitted synchronous scoring of real-time observations and computer data entry.

The BNBAS[31] was used to assess neonatal movement. The predominate states during BNBAS testing were noted along with two individual items of activity and lability of states. The activity score is a summary of the total activity of the neonate throughout the examination. The lability of states score reflects the number of state changes (over 15 seconds) within the exam period. The "organization processes: state control" cluster was used from the a priori clusters.[33] The state control cluster score is based on scores of habituation, predominant state, peak of excitement, lability of states, rapidity of build-up, irritability, and self-quieting items. Range of state and regulation of state were used from the 7-cluster scale.[34] Range of state is determined from the peak of excitement, rapidity of build-up, irritability, and lability of state items. Regulation of state is derived from the cuddliness, consolability, self-quieting, and hand-to-mouth items.

Procedure

After giving informed consent, participating women received serial ultrasound imagings at 12, 14 and 16 weeks of gestation. The imagings were conducted from 4-6 PM by a certified ultrasonographer.

Videotapes of the 305 minutes of imaging were scored using 100 frames-per-second analysis for frequency and duration of inactivity and activity. The whole tape was observed first in real-time and scored for usable and non-usable sections, as suggested by the Fetal-Posture and Movement System (F-PAM) described in this issue. Segments of movement or posture (inactivity) were scored next using frame-by-frame advance of the videotape. Only segments of several minutes duration were scored at any one session in order to prevent observer drift. The scoring procedure was developed after an extensive training period with 25-minute videotaped imagings of one pilot subject at 12, 14 and 16 weeks. Based on the pilot data, the authors established the following criteria for scoring categories of inactivity, activity, and tape usability.

1. Inactivity — no gross body movements. Fetus must exhibit for at least 5 seconds.
2. Activity — nearly continuous trunk and extremity multi-plane movements. Fetus must exhibit for 5 seconds to be termed activity.
3. Nonusable — over 50% of fetus not observed for over 4 seconds.

Scoring began at the start of a movement or inactive period and ended at the final complete movement or inactive period. When viewing was obscured for less than four seconds, and the code before and after were the same, the segment was termed usable. When a nonusable segment interfered with determination of an inactivity-activity cycle, that cycle was not included in the calculations of the median duration of activity per cycle. Inter-rater agreement was based on the percent of codes, within two seconds, that each researcher had in common with one other researcher.

Using these guidelines, the three raters achieved 86% inter-rater reliability on one pilot tape. After the four study imagings were scored, a random sample of 10 percent was rescored by a rater blind to study results. The percent of time the codes were the same was used as an additional measure of reliability. Following birth, the

BNBAS was conducted at 42 weeks corrected age by certified testers.

Analysis

Friedman's Rank Test for Correlated Samples[35] was used as the non-parametric test of choice to analyze the fetal movement data of four subjects at three ages. When significance ($p \leq .05$) was found, a Friedman's multiple comparison test was conducted to determine where the significance occurred. In a descriptive analysis, the frequency of inactivity-activity at 16 weeks was compared to the BNBAS state control, regulation of state, and range of state scores.

RESULTS

Researchers achieved adequate inter-rater reliability on precise analysis of videotapes of ultrasound imagings with lengthy training. The mean percentage of inter-rater agreement for the number of codes each observer had in agreement was 73.31 percent, while the mean percent for the amount of time in those codes was 89.72 percent (Table 1).

Fetal inactivity and activity were scored, not on the total 25 minutes of taping, but on the percent of tape that had a clear image and was able to be scored. The percent of usable tape for all subjects at the three ages ranged from 74.64 percent to 97.85 percent, with a mean of 91.51 percent.

Percent of total fetal activity decreased significantly from 12 to 16 weeks gestation ($X_F^2 = 8.00$). On post hoc analysis, the significant difference was from 14 to 16 weeks ($z_o = 6.14$). The increase in fetal activity from 12 to 14 weeks gestation was not significant (Figure 1).

The frequency of inactivity-activity cycles increased significantly from 12 to 16 weeks ($X_F^2 = 6.50$). Post hoc analysis showed no difference between 12 and 14 weeks or 14 and 16 weeks (Table 2). Although the frequency of cycles increased from 12 to 16 weeks, there was no significant change in duration of activity per cycle

Table 1. Inter-Rater Reliability for Three Raters
on Time and Codes

Raters	Time Agreement (%)	Code Agreement (%)
1 and 2	90.60	67.42
1 and 3	95.10	76.57
2 and 3	83.45	75.91
Mean	89.72	73.31

over the three gestational ages (Table 3). There was a positive trend indicating a decrease in duration of activity between 14 and 16 weeks.

Data on the BNBAS showed no clear differences among the infants (Table 4). State 5 was a predominate state for all subjects, and all were scored moderately active during testing. Newborn infants differed only on the BNBAS item of lability of state, and on regulation of state on the 7-cluster analysis. On the BNBAS lability of states, subjects 017 and 020 had fewer state changes (9-10) compared to subjects 018 and 019 who had 14-15. Full term subjects 018 and 020 neonatally had the highest scores on the regulation of state cluster from the BNBAS (Table 4), and at 16 weeks of gestation had the fewest cycle changes (Table 2) and the longest duration of activity (Table 3). Scores on regulation of state were variable. The low scores of subjects 017 and 019 were consistent with the a priori cluster analysis describing these newborns as "very labile." However, 020 whose score on regulation of state was the best, also rated a "very labile" designation on state control. Subjects 018 and 020 received moderate to moderately high scores on regulation of state and were classified by the investigators as the

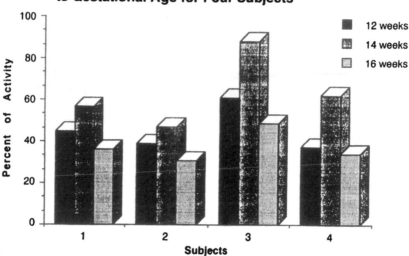

Figure 1 - Percent of Fetal Activity According to Gestational Age for Four Subjects*

*Friedman's nonparametic analysis of variance by ranks (df=2, p=0.05, x_F^2>5.99) was significant (x_F^2=8.00). The difference was between 14 and 16 weeks of gestation (zo=6.14).

most organized during the fetal period. These were the two full term pregnancies.

On the range of state scores, the lower the score the less optimal the behavior. Subject 019 received the lowest score (2.50) on this cluster compared to the other three subjects (3.50, 3.50, 3.80). Subject 019 as a fetus received the highest activity score at all three gestational ages (Figure 1), the greatest frequency of inactivity-activity cycles at 16 weeks (Table 2), and the smallest duration of movement at 16 weeks (Table 3). Subject 019 was the earliest born of the four subjects at 35 weeks of gestation. Subject 017, born at 37 weeks of gestation, received the next highest fetal activity score (Figure 1) and frequency of fetal inactivity-activity cycles (Table 2), and the next smallest duration of movement at 16 weeks (Table 3).

Table 2.   Frequency of Rest-Activity Cycles Per Minute at 12, 14, 16 Weeks for Four Subjects*

Subjects	Gestational Age		
	12 WEEKS	14 WEEKS	16 WEEKS
017	.78	1.12	1.51
018	.83	.90	1.06
019	.53	.54	1.54
020	.92	.54	.96
Mean	.77	.78	1.27

*Friedman's nonparametric analysis of variance by ranks (df=2, p=0.05, $X_F^2 > 5.99$) was significant ($X_F^2 = 6.50$). A multiple comparison for Friedman's showed a significant difference (Zo=6.14) between 12 and 16 weeks gestation.

DISCUSSION

The achievement of relatively good reliability on precise scoring of fetal movement from observation was a major result when compared with the reliability reported from other studies. The achievement of adequate interrater reliability is a first step in the psychometrically appropriate measurement of fetal movement. The reliability discrepancy between the percent of codes and duration of codes was due to the limitation the investigators placed on themselves in identifying a code within a 2-second time frame.

A further factor related to the replication and comparison of study results is the description of the amount of tape that was usable, i.e., able to be scored. Among previous studies, Swartjes et al.[26] is one of

Table 3.   Mean Duration (seconds) of Activity Per Cycle
at Three   Gestational Ages for Four Subjects*

Subjects	Gestational Age		
	12-WEEKS	14-WEEKS	16-WEEKS
017	17.56	17.23	7.93
018	16.74	24.00	12.73
019	37.97	20.73	7.79
020	6.70	17.74	10.62
Mean	19.74	19.93	9.77

*Friedman's non-parametric analysis of variance by ranks
(df=2, p=0.05, $X_F^2>5.99$) showed no significant difference
($X_F^2=3.50$) between weeks on durations of activity. When
isolating 14 and 16 weeks (df=1, p=0.05, $X_F^2>3.84$), there
was a significant difference ($X_F^2=4$).

the only groups that has revealed that the percent of usable tape may be as low as 70 percent. Precise three-dimensional movements are difficult to see throughout an entire tape using two-dimensional technology. Movement may be lost if the transducer remains stationery, or transducer movement interferes with clear imaging as it follows the fetus moving in and across different planes.

From our preliminary data on low-risk pregnant women, and data from deVries, Visser and Prechtl,[8,20] we hypothesized that there would be a decrease in movement from 14 to 16 weeks. In this study, the decrease in fetal movement from 14 to 16 weeks was significant. Animal research suggests that several processes in the

Table 4. Neonatal Behavior at Corrected Age of 2 Weeks
          According to the Brazelton Neonatal Behavioral
          Assessment Scale (BNBAS)

BNBAS Categories	Subjects			
	017 (37 weeks)	018 (40 weeks)	019 (35 weeks)	020 (40 weeks)
Predominate State	5,6	2,5	5,6	4,5
Activity	5 Moderate	6 Mod. to Much	6 Mod. to Much	5 Moderate
Lability of States	4	6	6	4
Regulation of State Seven-cluster	3.80 Low	5.50 Moderate	3.75 Low	6.50 Moderate
State Control Four-cluster	3 Very labile	2 Normal	3 Very labile	3 Very labile
Range of State Seven-cluster	3.80	3.50	2.50	3.50

developing nervous system occur at about this time in gestation. These explanations may not be valid in describing our results, but it appears worthy of conjecture whether we are observing the clinical effects of neuronal cell death[36,37] or selective disintegration of neural synapses,[38] or migration of neurons.[39] A large subject pool would be needed to address this question.

The frequency of inactivity-activity units increased significantly from 12 to 16 weeks. These results suggest that 12 to 16 weeks may be a transition period in which all movements are being expressed, as suggested by the deVries group, but their organization into characteristic patterns and cycles is incomplete. Support for this idea comes from Japan.[40] In a recent study, the frequency and duration of fetal activity reportedly decreased, while the frequency and duration of inactivity increased from 14 weeks, plateauing at 37 weeks.

The possible relationship between fetal and neonatal behavior is preliminary, and the use of only four subjects limits the generalizability of this finding. The clinical perception of the investigators that 018 and 020 were more organized fetuses was somewhat supported at neonatal testing. That 019 as a fetus and neonate was the least organized provides incentive for further study of individual differences and developmental continuity, but prematurity could have been a factor here. Individual consistencies in movement have been noted in previous descriptions of fetal general movements.[30] Future study might incorporate a comparison of the increased frequency of cycles at 16 weeks gestation to the increased lability and decreased regulation of state (017, 019) observed neonatally.

A major study limitation relates to the small number of subjects. Because of the intensive nature of observing and accurately scoring the imagings, a large subject pool is impractical. We have decided to observe rigorously a small number of subjects by analyzing the movements frame-by-frame, rather than real-time.

The two-dimensional nature of obstetric imaging presented a problem, in addition, by limiting the amount of usable tape available for analysis. In this study, almost 25 percent less tape was scored for one subject at 16 weeks, limiting comparison across subjects. The Committee on the Protection of the Rights of Human Subjects limited imaging to 25 minutes, a time which often is used in diagnostic obstetric imaging. Studies in Europe have used 1-2 hours of imaging. Even with longer imaging durations, investigators assume that they are analyzing representative samples of a 24-hour day. Only Nasello-Patterson et al.[21] in Canada have been permitted that duration of imaging.

A second testing on the BNBAS on the next day might have provided more valid neonatal data. The BNBAS testing was done in the home at the child's corrected age of two weeks, permitting the certified examiner to initiate testing with the child asleep and between feedings.

FUTURE STUDY

The intent of this study was to increase knowledge about periods of inactivity and activity of the young fetus. Further study is needed with more subjects to determine the developmental sequence of these periods and the early coincidence of state parameters. This knowledge may enable researchers to differentiate those fetuses at risk or in need of intervention from low-risk fetuses.

Specifically, we need to clarify an apparent intermediate category of inactivity with incidental gross body movements lasting less than 5 seconds. On preliminary review of additional imagings, this category consistently appears and may offer additional information related to underlying neural mechanisms. Factors such as this one may be critical as we initiate study of cocaine-exposed fetuses and fetuses of diabetic mothers.

The continued exploration of developmental continuity and individual differences requires use of the same assessment instrument or of instruments assessing the same domains. The BNBAS is not measuring the same domains as were observed in utero. Further development of the F-PAM and the Q-MOVE will permit its use with newborn infants.

REFERENCES

1. Arduini D, Rizzo G, Giorlandino C, Dell'Aqua S, Valensise H, Romanini C. The development of fetal behavioral states: a longitudinal study. *Prenat Diagn.* 1986; 6:117-124.

2. Visser GHA, Poelmann-Weesjes G, Cohen TMN, Bekedam DJ. Fetal behavior at 30 to 32 weeks of gestation. *Pediatr Res.* 1987; 22(6):655-658.

3. Swartjes JM, vanGeijn HP, Mantel R, vanWoerden EE, Schoemaker HC. Coincidence of behavioral state parameters in the human fetus at three gestational ages. *Early Hum Dev.* 1990; 23:75-83.

4. Arduini D, Rizzo G, Massacesi M, Romanini C, Mancuso S. Longitudinal assessment of behavioral transitions in healthy human fetuses during the third trimester of pregnancy. *J Perinat Med.* 1991; 19:67-72.

5. Drogtrop AP, Ubels R, Nijhuis JG. The association between fetal body movements, eye movements and heart rate patterns in pregnancies between 25 and 30 weeks of gestation. *Early Hum Dev.* 1990; 23:67-73.

6. Ianniruberto A, Tajani E. Ultrasonographic study of fetal movements. *Semin Perinatol.* 1981; 5:175-181.

7. Milani Comparetti A. The neurophysiologic and clinical implications of studies on fetal motor behavior. *Semin Perinat.* 1981; 5(2):183-189.

8. deVries JIP, Visser GHA, Prechtl HFR. The emergence of fetal behavior. I. Qualitative aspects. *Early Human Dev.* 1982; 7:301-322.

9. Schulte FJ, Michaelis R, Nolte R, Albert A, Parl U, Lasson U. Brain and behavioural maturation in newborn infants of diabetic mothers. Part I:Nerve conduction and EEG patterns. *Neuropaediatrie.* 1969; 1:24-35.

10. Birnholz JC. The development of human fetal eye movement patterns. *Science.* 1981; 213:679-681.

11. Martin CB. Assessment of fetal well being with observation of different fetal movement types. *J Perinatal Med.* 1984; 12:26-28.

12. Sakata H. A clinical evaluation of fetal well being based on fetal behavior with emphasis on conditions contributing to the dissociation of behavior. *Nippon-Sanka-Fujinka-Gakkai-Zasshi (English abstract).* 1991; 43(8):853-863.

13. van Geijn HP, Jongsma HW, de Haan J, Eskes TKAB, Prechtl HFR. Heart rate as indicator of the behavioral state: studies in the newborn infant and prospects for fetal heart monitoring. *Am J Obstet Gynecol.* 1980; 136:1061-1066.

14. Nijuis JG, Prechtl HFR, Martin CB Jr, Bots RSGM. Are there behavioral states in the human fetus? *Early Hum Dev.* 1982; 6:177-195.

15. Prechtl HFR, Nijhuis JG. Eye movements in the human fetus and newborn. *Behav Brain Res.* 1983; 10:119-124.

16. Moore KL. *Before We Are Born,* 3rd ed. Philadelphia: W.B.Saunders; 1989:52.

17. Gagnon R, Campbell K, Hunse C, Patrick J. Patterns of human fetal heart rate accelerations from 26 weeks to term. *Am J Obstet Gynecol.* 1987; 157: 743-748.

18. Sparling JW, Wilhelm IJ: The qualitative assessment of fetal arm movements. *Phys Ther.* 1989; 69:397.

19. Roodenburg PJ, Wladimiroff JW, vanEs A, Prechtl HFR. Classification and quantitative aspects of fetal movements during the second half of normal pregnancy. *Early Hum Dev.* 1991; 25:19-35.

20. deVries JIP, Visser GHA, Prechtl HFR. The emergence of fetal behaviour. II. Quantitative aspects. *Early Hum Dev.* 1985; 12:99-120.

21. Nasello-Paterson C, Natale R, Connors G. Ultrasonic evaluation of fetal body movements over twenty-four hours in the human fetus at twenty-four to twenty-eight weeks' gestation. *Am J Obstet Gynecol.* 1988; 158:312-316.

22. deVries JIP, Visser GHA, Mulder EJH, Prechtl HFR. Diurnal and other variations in fetal movement and heart rate pattern at 20 to 22 weeks. *Early Hum Dev.* 1987; 15:333-348.

23. Pillai M, James D. Hiccups and breathing in human fetuses. *Arch Dis Child.* 1990; 65:1072-1075.

24. Bekedam DJ, Visser GHA, deVries JJ, Prechtl HFR. Motor behavior in the growth retarded fetus. *Early Hum Dev.* 1985; 12:155-165.

25. Prechtl HFR. Fetal behavior. *European Journal of Obstetrical, Gynecological and Reproductive Biology.* 1989; 32-33.

26. Swartjes JM, vanGeijn HP, Meinardi H, vanAlphen M, Schoemaker HC. Fetal rest-activity cycles and chronic exposure to antiepileptic drugs. *Epilepsia.* 1991; 32(5):722-728.

27. Rizzo G, Arduini D, Pennestri F, Romanini C, Mancuso S. Fetal behavior in growth retardation: its relationship to fetal blood flow. *Prenatal Diag.* 1987; 7:229-238.

28. Ardiuni D, Rizzo G, Caforio L, Romanini C, Mancuso S. The development of behavioral states in hydrocephalic fetuses. *Fetal Ther.* 1987;2:135-141.

29. Robertson SS. Human cyclic motility: fetal-newborn continuities and newborn state differences. *Dev Psychobiol.* 1987;20:425-442.

30. deVries JIP, Visser GHA, Prechtl HFR. The emergence of fetal behaviour. III. individual differences and consistencies. *Early Hum Dev.* 1988;16:85-103.

31. Brazelton TB. *Neonatal Behavioral Assessment Scale*, ed 2. London: Spastics International Medical Publications; 1984.

32. Szostek TK. *Observational Coding System.* Research Triangle Park, NC: Research Triangle Collaborative, Inc.; 1988.

33. Als H, Tronic E, Lester BM, Brazelton TB. The Brazelton Neonatal Behavioral Assessment Scale (BNBAS). *J Abn Child Psychol.* 1977;5:215-237.

34. Lester BM. Change and stability in neonatal behavior. In: Brazelton TB, Lester BM. *New Approaches to Developmental Screening of Infants.* New York, NY: Elsevier Science Publishing Co.; 1983:51-75.

35. Howell DC. *Statistical Method for Psychology.* Boston, MA: Duxbury Press; 1982:508-510.

36. Hirsch HVB, Jacobson M. The perfectible brain: Principles of neuronal development. In: Gazzaniga MS, Blakemore C, eds. *Handbook of Psychobiology.* New York, NY: Academic Press; 1975.

37. Mole R. Possible hazards of imaging and Doppler ultrasound in obstetrics. *Birth.* 1986; 13:23-32.

38. Purves D, Lichtman JW. Elimination of synapses in the developing nervous system. *Science.* 1980; 210:153-157.

39. Ziskin MC, Petitti DB. Epidemiology of human exposure to ultrasound: a critical review. *Ultrasound Med Biol.* 1988; 14(2):91-96.

40. Tatsumura M. Studies on features of fetal movement and development of human fetus with use of fetal actogram. *Nippon-Sanka-Fujinka-Gakkai-Zasshi (English abstract).* 1991; 43(9):864-873.

Kinematic Study
of Human Fetal Shoulder Movement
in Utero:
Preliminary Results

J. Audrey Macdonald
E.A. Lyons

SUMMARY. This paper describes the methodology used for a kinematic study of human fetal shoulder movement in utero. The data obtained in routine ultrasound examinations was recorded on videotape for repeated playback and motion analysis. Preliminary findings are presented for four subjects, one of whom may have experienced less than optimal conditions in utero. Findings were charted on a Fetal Movement Time Line, and are discussed in relation to normal motor development.

With technological refinement of diagnostic ultrasound, a shift has occurred in fetal study from an emphasis on anatomical components to an investigation of the complex neurobehaviour and physi-

J. Audrey Macdonald, PT, is Assistant Professor in the Division of Physiotherapy, School of Medical Rehabilitation, University of Manitoba. E.A. Lyons, MD, is Professor and Head of the Department of Radiology, University of Manitoba, Head of the Department of Radiology, Health Sciences Center, Associate Professor in the Department of Anatomy, University of Manitoba.

This study is being carried out in partial fulfillment of requirements for MSc degree in Anatomy and has been supported by the School of Medical Rehabilitation and the Department of Radiology, University of Manitoba.

The authors would like to acknowledge Mr. C. Harrington, RT(NM), RDMS, Clinical Instructor, Section of Ultrasound, Health Sciences Centre, for performing the ultrasound scans on all subjects and the Department of Obstetrics at Manitoba Clinic, especially Dr. C.K. Yuen.

181

ology of the fetus.[1] One of the most significant advances provided by ultrasound has been the potential it offers to examine the spatial and temporal characteristics of the movement of fetuses in their natural environment. Observation of these characteristics enables us to speculate as to their significance.

Fetal and infant movement have been described as a developmental continuum,[2] with structural development related to functional movement.[3] Because normal and abnormal movement patterns undergo qualitative changes with postnatal maturation, it seems reasonable to ask whether movement progresses in a similar manner prenatally. Previous studies have suggested that changes in the quality of movement will precede changes in the quantitative output of motility in the compromised fetus.[4] Thus, the study of the spatial and temporal characteristics of fetal movement could significantly improve our understanding of neonatal sensorimotor functioning and the evolution of congenital motor disabilities.

The rapid rate of early neuromuscular development, and the interweaving of structural with motor development are well-known characteristics of postnatal development. These same factors and relationships can be observed in prenatal development. In the upper extremity, for example, bilateral shoulder flexion and extension have been observed at eight weeks, two weeks before rotation of the limb buds,[5] and rotation at the glenohumeral joint has been noted at nine weeks,[5] a week-and-a-half prior to the beginning of joint cavitation. These observations suggest the need to study more precisely the movement of the glenohumeral joint.

The purpose of this pilot study, therefore, was to investigate scapulohumeral posture and abduction/adduction movement in four low-risk fetuses at 20 weeks of gestation. The specific objectives of the study were to determine: the feasibility of collecting kinematic data from fetal scapular and humeral movements; the posture of the glenohumeral joint during inactivity; the ranges of motion, duration, and velocity of spontaneous abduction and adduction movements at the glenohumeral joint; and the relative contribution of scapular movement to each of these movements.

SHOULDER DEVELOPMENT

Previous studies have shown that upper extremity movement occurs frequently during the first half of gestation. Birnholz[4] identified five, and Ianniruberto and Tajani[6] noted eight, specific movement patterns that involved the upper extremity and were present by 16 weeks of gestation. deVries et al.[5] described seven movement patterns involving the upper extremity that were present by 11 weeks, and found that the incidence of isolated arm movements gradually increased from 8 through 19 weeks.[7] Glenohumeral abduction and adduction were among the fetal repertoire.[5] Highlights in the early development of the glenohumeral joint are described in Table 1 and range from the appearance of the limb bud at 5.5 weeks,[8] to the presence of functional hand-to-mouth movements at 9.5 weeks[5] and alternating arm movements at 13 weeks.[6]

METHODOLOGY

Subjects

Four maternal volunteers were recruited through the offices of private obstetricians and provided informed consent before being enrolled in the study. Maternal subjects ranged in age from 24 to 31 years, were known to be carrying less than a 12-week, low-risk, singleton fetus, worked outside the home, and were for the most part not involved in strenuous activities outside of work. This was the first pregnancy for three of the four women. One subject (subject B) had eight previous spontaneous abortions. Her only living child was born at 28 weeks after abrupt onset of labor. The women were not substance abusers, had negligible daily caffeine intake, and none were taking any medication beyond nutritional supplements. One subject (C) smoked. The obstetrician anticipated no major complications for any pregnancy.

Data on fetal subjects is shown in Table 2. The course of pregnancy is noted along with pertinent birth data. Results of the follow-up gross motor assessment of the fetal subjects to 4-12 months of age are described.

Table 1. Highlights in Early Development of the Glenohumeral Joint

Age in Post Menstrual Weeks	Structures Identified and Movements Observed	Investigator and Year	Methodology and Documentation
5.5	Upper limb bud.	O'Rahilly & Muller[3], 1987	Embryological study of 17 specimens.
6.5	Scapula at level of C4.	Lewis[4], 1902	Embryological study of 4 specimens.
7	Premuscle masses of shoulder girdle. Brachial plexus divisions. Humerus has head, shaft, condyles. Scapula has coracoid and acromion. Coracoclavicular ligament.	Lewis[4], 1902	Embryological study of 4 specimens.
7.5	Coracoacromial and transverse scapular ligaments, tendon of long head of biceps. Deltoid, supraspinatus, infraspinatus, teres minor, subscapularis, teres major, latissimus dorsi muscles.	Lewis[4], 1902	Embryological study of 4 specimens.
	Contralateral neck and trunk side flexion, including action of upper trapezius.	Hooker[5], 1952	Stimulation of 2 exteriorized fetuses with light moving touch to the perioral area. Recorded in photographs.

8	Scapula between C8 and T5. Shoulder girdle muscles have established scapular attachments.	Lewis[4], 1902	Embryological study of 4 specimens.
	Scapula has neck and glenoid.	Gardner & Gray[6], 1953	Embryological study of several specimens.
	Sometimes slight limb movements during vermicular movements.	Ianniruberto & Tajani, 1981	Ultrasound observation of spontaneous movement in utero of 82 or more fetuses.
	Startle, including bilateral shoulder extension or flexion.	deVries[8], 1982	Prolonged ultrasound observation of spontaneous movement in utero of 11 fetuses. Recorded on videotape.
8.5	Contralateral and ipsilateral neck and trunk side flexion, both including bilateral shoulder extension.	Hooker[5], 1952	Stimulation of 6 exteriorized fetuses with light moving touch to the perioral area. Recorded in photographs.
9	Glenoid labrum.	Gardner & Gray[6], 1953	Embryological study of several specimens.

TABLE 1 (continued)

Age in Post Menstrual Weeks	Structures Identified and Movements Observed	Investigator and Year	Methodology and Documentation
	Triceps muscle. Suprascapular and coracohumeral ligaments. Long head of biceps in bicipital groove.	Lewis[4], 1902	Embryological study of 4 specimens.
	Isolated arm movements, including shoulder flexion, extension, abduction, adduction, internal rotation, external rotation.	deVries[8], 1982	Prolonged ultrasound observation of spontaneous movement in utero of 11 fetuses. Recorded on videotape.
9.5	Shoulder flexion.	Hooker[5], 1952	Stimulation of uncertain number of exteriorized fetuses with proprioceptive input to fingers. Recorded in photographs.
	Hand-face contact. Stretch, including bilateral elevation of arms above head and shoulder external rotation.	deVries[8], 1982	Prolonged ultrasound observation of spontaneous movement in utero of 11 fetuses. Recorded on videotape.
10	Limb bud has rotated.	O'Rahilly & Gardner, 1975	Embryological study of uncertain number of embryos.

10.5	Scapula has spine. Humerus has neck, greater and lesser tuberosities. Joint cavitation beginning. Glenohumeral ligaments.	Gardner & Gray[6], 1953	Embryological study of several specimens.
11.5	Bilateral shoulder medial rotation accompanying trunk extension.	Hooker[5], 1952	Stimulation of uncertain number of exteriorized fetuses with light moving touch to midline of face. Recorded in photographs.
	Shoulder abduction.	Hooker[5], 1952	Stimulation of uncertain number of exteriorized fetuses with light moving touch to any of upper extremity or upper chest. Recorded in photographs.
12	Joint capsule regionally differentiated.	Gardner & Gray[6], 1953	Embryological study of several specimens.
13	Creeping and climbing movements.	Ianniruberto & Tajani, 1981	Ultrasound observation of spontaneous movement in utero of 82 or more fetuses.

Table 2. Subject Characteristics

Subjects	Maternal Age and History*	Course of this Pregnancy	Delivery & Gender	Birth Weight	Apgar Score	Gross Motor Scores on ABC
A	27 years, G_1P_0	uncomplicated	spontaneous at 40 wk., F	7 lb., 15 oz.	10, 10	1 year at age 1 year
B	31 years, $G_2P_1A_8$	14 weeks-choroid plexus cysts 2 mm. diameter, resolved at 30 weeks. 28 weeks-minor abruption	induced at 38 wk., M	7 lb., 3 oz.	9, 10	4 months at age 4 months (corrected age 3.5 months)
C	24 years, G_1P_0	16 weeks-dilated renal collecting tubules, resolved at 36 weeks	spontaneous at 40 wk., M	8 lb., 6 oz.	10, 10	9-10 months at age 10 months
D	27 years G_1P_0	12 weeks to 20 weeks-fetal measurements subnormal on US. 20 weeks asymmetric intrauterine growth retardation, gestational diabetes. 24 weeks hypertension.	Cesarean at 32 wk. due to drop in maternal platelet count, M	3 lb., 1 oz.	3, 8	11-12 months at 1 year (corrected age 10 months)

*G = Gravida
 P = Parity
 A = Spontaneous Abortion

Instrumentation

The Ultramark 9 (ATL, Bothwell, WA) machine with a curved linear array transducer was used by a certified ultrasonographer. The frequency was 3.5 MHz, and the output was kept at the minimum necessary to produce a diagnostic quality of image. Ultrasound images are magnified in ultrasound scans, so the internal measuring scale of the ultrasound machine was checked with an external measuring device, a ruler, for accuracy. For data observation, a high-resolution monitor with freeze-frame and single-frame advance capabilities was used.

Follow-up postnatal gross motor evaluation was conducted using the Assessment of Behavioral Components (ABC).[12] This instrument was developed to assess the motor behaviors of children with cerebral palsy. The 92 criterion-referenced test items provide finely graded increments for assessing postural tone and range of motion (17), reflex activity (10), and active movement patterns (65 items). Interrater reliability on assessment of 70 children averaged in the 90 percent range. Test-retest reliability was over 85 percent.

Procedure

Data Collection. At 20 weeks of gestation, each subject received a ten-minute ultrasound scan that was performed in the routine manner with a full bladder and the subject positioned in supine. All scans were carried out in the early afternoon by the same sonographer. All four fetuses were in sidelying posture, and each scan began with the recording of fetal biparietal diameter and femoral length. The fetal shoulder nearest the transducer was then scanned in a longitudinal section, in the plane of the scapula, for approximately eight minutes. Every attempt was made to keep the ipsilateral scapula and humerus in the plane of section, even through any changes in fetal position. The image was recorded onto VHS videotape for later analysis.

Data Reduction. A second-generation videotape was made with a time code and a 30-frame per second frame count. Each videotape was played back repeatedly for analysis. Precision of angular measurements was enhanced by having the video screen directly at eye level. The fetal starting position, and its relation to the line of gravity, was traced onto a transparency at the beginning of the tape and any time the position changed. The visibility of scapula and humerus was noted for each frame of videotape. Each movement of the humerus was identified in anatomical terms (as described in Table 3) and its duration measured.

The relative scapulohumeral angle (GIPD), as shown in Figure 1, was measured with a protractor (resolution = 1 degree) on the still video screen for its inactive posture, as well as in each of the 30 frames/second for each movement. The absolute angle of the humerus (PD) and the absolute angle of the lateral border of the scapula (GI) were measured with the protractor from the right horizontal in each frame of each movement. This horizontal line was

Table 3.   Movement Specifications

Movement	Each change in direction of movement of humerus is considered a new movement. Continued movement of the humerus in the same direction is considered a new movement after there has been no apparent motion for 2 or more video frames.
Abduction/ Adduction of Humerus	Movements occurring in the plane of the scapula,[13] because diagnostic ultrasound allows observation in only one plane.
Horizontal Adduction/ Abduction	Movements occurring in the transverse plane, with respect to the fetus.
Flexion/ Extension of Humerus	Movements occurring within the sagittal plane.[13] The movements can be incompletely viewed in this plane.
Elevation/ Depression of Scapula	Translatory motion of scapula occurring cephalad or caudally along the ribcage.[13]
Abduction/ Adduction of Scapula	Translatory motion of scapula occurring along the ribcage, away from/toward vertebral column.[13]
Upward/ Downward Rotation of Scapula	Rotary motions of scapula in which the glenoid fossa tilted upward or downward.[13]

FIGURE 1. Posterior View of Scapula and Humerus*

* The small size of the fetus allows concurrent observation of the scapula and humerus when the humerus lies within the same plane as the scapula. Angle GI, measured from the right horizontal, is the absolute angle of the lateral border of scapula. Angle PD, measured from the right horizontal, is the absolute angle of the humerus. The relative angle, GIPD, is the angle between the long axis of the lateral border of the scapula and the long axis of the humerus.

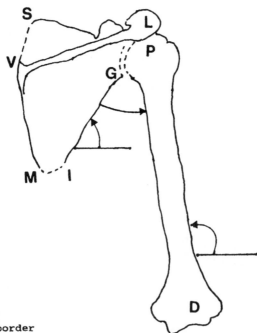

```
VM - medial border

SL = superior border

GI = long axis of lateral border

PD = long axis of humerus

___ = incompletely visualized
```

previously established with respect to the horizontal of the video monitor. The length of the humerus (PD) was measured with a ruler (resolution = 1 millimeter) in each frame of each movement. To determine the net movement of the scapula, the extreme limits of the superior and lateral borders of the scapula were traced onto a transparency applied over the video screen in the initial and final frames of each movement, as shown in Figure 2. The location of any visible reference point (p) on the thoracic spine was also

FIGURE 2. Measurement of the Net Movement of the Scapula*

* The actual distance from m (midpoint of initial line SL) to m' (midpoint of final line S′L′), measured on the transparency with a ruler is the net movement of the scapula. The reference point on the thoracic spine is p.

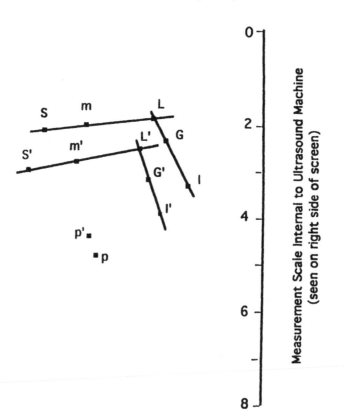

marked onto the transparency in the initial and final frames of each movement.

Data Analysis. The inactive postures are the relative scapulo-humeral angles (GIPD) measured during each period of time without movement. Movements of the humerus were quantified in degrees of range of motion as measured at the relative angle, and the difference between initial and final video frames. Any movement of the humerus out of the plane of the scapula was determined by comparing the initial and final measurements of humeral length (PD). The angular velocity of the movement was determined by calculating the number of degrees of change in the absolute angle of the humerus (PD) per second.

Net movement of the scapula was determined on the transparency by joining points S and L, and G and I, to create lines SL and GI for both the initial and final positions of the scapula, as shown in Figure 2. The superior/inferior distance and medial/lateral distance travelled by the midpoint (m) of the line SL was measured against the internal scale of the ultrasound machine, to determine elevation/depression and abduction/adduction of the scapula on the chest wall. Any distance between the initial and final locations of the external reference point (p) was similarly measured, in order to determine whether apparent movement of the scapula was actually movement of the thorax. The difference in angle between the initial line SL and the final line SL was measured with a protractor to determine the net upward/downward rotation of the scapula on the chest wall.

The more specific scapular rotation accompanying each frame of humeral motion was obtained by comparing the absolute angles of scapula and humerus with the relative angle, in order to determine the relative contribution of each bone to the movement.

Construction of Fetal Movement Time Line. The Fetal Movement Time Line was constructed from the written log of the frame-by-frame analysis of the videotape as shown in Figure 3. Each movement of the humerus is noted along the humerus (h) line for its duration of time in video frames. Movements of the humerus into flexion, abduction, horizontal adduction, or external rotation are indicated above the line; extension, adduction, horizontal abduction, or internal rotation are indicated below the line. These designations were made based on proprioceptive neuromuscular facilita-

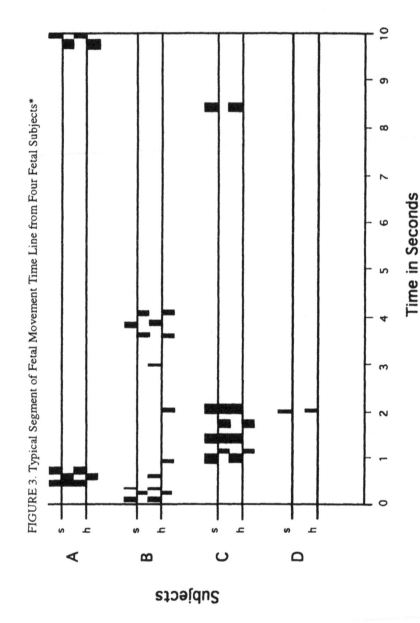

FIGURE 3. Typical Segment of Fetal Movement Time Line from Four Fetal Subjects*

Time in Seconds

* Scapular movement is simultaneously marked above and below the line indicating the expected combination of movement components, e.g., elevation with downward rotation.

tion patterns (PNF) and on previous observation of fetal shoulder movements. The height of the block for each movement is uniform, so does not relate to its range of motion or speed. The direction of net scapular movement accompanying each humeral movement is recorded along the scapula line (s) of the Fetal Movement Time Line. Upward rotation, elevation, and abduction of the scapula are recorded above the line; downward rotation, depression, and adduction are recorded below the line.

Reliability. Intra-observer reliability was determined for these four cases by repeated testing after a two-week interval on Subject C, selected because it was the most difficult tape to analyze due to the frequent body movements. The magnitude of error found was 0.45 degrees (SD = 0.79 degrees) for the GIPD angles; 0.55 degrees (SD = 1.03) for the GI angle, and 0.57 (SD = 1.21) for the PD angle.

Follow-Up. Subjects are being followed postnatally until corrected age of two years. Gross motor development is assessed quarterly, using the ABC.

RESULTS

Practicality of Data Collection

From the initial eight minutes of videotape, the amount of tape in which the scapula and humerus were simultaneously visible was approximately 6 minutes for subject A (74.9%) and subject C (78.1%), 4.6 minutes (57.4%) for subject B, and 6.9 minutes (84.5%) for subject D. The shoulder movements were usually short in duration, however, so the amount of tape actually showing movements ranged from approximately 1 percent (1.1% for C, 0.8% for B) to 0.1 percent (0.3% for A, 0.17% for D).

Inactive Postures

The inactive shoulder posture changed 10 times for A, 58 times for B, 65 times for C, and 14 times for D. In all four subjects, the majority of changes in inactive posture occurred after disappearance of the humerus, suggesting that further movements occurred while out of transducer view. D's mean inactive posture was the most adducted (21.5 degrees) when compared with subject A (33.4 degrees), subject B (40.7 degrees), and subject C (56.1 degrees), and D's range of inactive postures covered only 51 degrees, compared with 167 degrees for A, 147 degrees for B, and 162 degrees for C.

Movement Characteristics

Table 4 summarizes the major characteristics of movements observed. There appears to be a wide range of movements with large standard deviations. A similarity was noted in the number of abduction and adduction movements for each subject. Besides abduction/ adduction movements, subject B demonstrated 17 movements of horizontal adduction/horizontal abduction, and subject D had one movement observed into flexion. Subject D, however, did not perform any adduction movements.

The scapular components of the abduction/adduction movements could be identified 43 times. The percent of humeral abduction and adduction in which specific scapular movements occurred is shown in Table 5. In all subjects, scapular abduction occurred with humeral abduction at least half of the time as anticipated, but in one subject, scapular abduction occurred with humeral adduction 75 percent of the time, a result inconsistent with adult glenohumeral rhythm. The ratio of scapular rotation to humeral movement was inconsistent with adult glenohumeral rhythm. In subject A, for example, 50 percent of the movements were characterized by a 1:1 ratio of scapular rotation to humeral movement, and 50 percent were characterized by a 5:1 ratio, both of which were different than in adult movement. Scapular analysis could not be carried out for eight movements or 18.6 percent of the movements observed because of shifts in plane.

Fetal Movement Time Line

Figure 3 depicts a typical ten-second segment of the Fetal Movement Time Line from each of the four cases. Subjects A, B, and C show a similar clustering of movement occurrences, each cluster consisting of several smooth, quick reversals of movement direc-

Table 4.   Characteristics of Shoulder Movements Observed Within
Eight Minutes for Four Subjects at 20 Weeks of Gestation

		Subjects			
		A	B	C	D
Characteristics					
Number					
Abduction		7	4	15	2
Adduction		8	2	13	0
Other		0	17	0	1
Duration (secs.)					
Abduction	Mean	0.11	0.27	0.20	0.27
	SD	0.02	0.42	0.23	0.19
Adduction	Mean	0.10	0.05	0.14	0.00
	SD	0.06	0.02	0.16	0.00
Range of Motion (degrees)					
Abduction	Mean	8.60	31.50	18.30	19.50
	SD	2.51	47.20	20.70	13.40
Adduction	Mean	6.30	10.50	13.70	0.00
	SD	2.90	4.90	16.90	0.00
Starting Angle (degrees)					
Abduction	Mean	30.60	46.80	24.90	8.00
	SD	11.60	16.50	28.00	7.10
Adduction	Mean	33.30	68.50	43.10	0.00
	SD	15.70	7.80	47.20	0.00
Peak Velocity (degrees/sec)					
Abduction	Mean	174.00	120.00	182.00	210.00
	SD	90.90	79.40	82.90	84.90
Adduction	Mean	125.00	255.00	152.00	0
	SD	91.80	63.60	64.20	0

tion. The mean length of each activity burst varied from 0.3
second (A) to 4.3 seconds (C). The mean length of periods without shoulder movements varied from 1.8 seconds (B) to 19.8
seconds (C). In subject D, there was movement in only one direction, the movements were of very short duration, and were separated by long periods (mean = 38.9 seconds) in which no movement occurred.

Table 5. Elements of Glenohumeral Rhythm Observed Over Eight
Minutes for Four Subjects (A, B, C, D) at 20 Weeks of Gestation
According to Percent of Humeral Abduction and Adduction in Which
Scapular Movements Occurred

Scapular Motion	Humeral Motion	
	ABDUCTION	ADDUCTION
Elevation	A = 100	A = 0
	B = 100	B = 0
	C = 60	C = 58*
	D = 0	D = 0
Depression	A = 0	A = 100
	B = 0	B = 0
	C = 40*	C = 42
	D = 100*	D = 0
Abduction	A = 100	A = 0
	B = 50	B = 0
	C = 60	C = 75*
	D = 50	D = 0
Adduction	A = 0	A = 0
	B = 50*	B = 0
	C = 40*	C = 25
	D = 50*	D = 0
Net Upward Rotation of Scapula	A = 40	A = 17*
	B = 100	B = 0
	C = 60	C = 31*
	D = 100	D = 0
Net Downward Rotation of Scapula	A = 40*	A = 60
	B = 0	B = 100
	C = 33*	C = 69
	D = 0	D = 0
Ratio of Scapular Rotation to Humeral Movement	A = 50 1:1*	A = 67 2:1*
	50 5:1*	33 1:2
	B = 50 1:3*	B = 100 1:1*
	50 1:4*	
	C = 67 1:3*	C = 22 1:4*
	11 1:12*	22 1:1*
	22 1:2	56 1:2
	D = 50 2:1*	D = 0
	50 1:1*	
Oscillation of Scapula**	A = 40	A = 17
	B = 100	B = 0
	C = 27	C = 23
	D = 100	D = 0

Scapular	Humeral Motion			
Motion	ABDUCTION		ADDUCTION	
No Scapula	A =	20	A =	33
Rotation	B =	0	B =	0
	C =	7	C =	0
	D =	0	D =	0

* Observations inconsistent with adult scapulohumeral rhythm.

** Rocking of scapula back and forth, into upward and downward rotation.

Follow-Up

These subjects have been followed postnatally for between 4 months (B) and 1 year (A and D), and gross motor development appears to be normal as determined by developmental assessment and parent report.

DISCUSSION

Feasibility

Kinematic measurements can be made on the videotape, as long as the image is clear enough. Clarity of the image can be improved somewhat by increasing the intensity of output and by choosing slender subjects. Of the tapes made in this study, 57-84 percent were useable, with one percent of the tapes useable for scapular and humerus movements. The length of ultrasound imaging for this study was not uncomfortable for the maternal subjects, and usually provided a sufficient number of movements for analysis. In subject B, there was considerable loss of simultaneous visualization due to movements occurring in the transverse plane; however, considerable information could be obtained as the humerus moved in and out of the plane of section. In instances where movements are less frequent, however, as in subject D, it may be desirable to continue scanning for at least eight minutes.

Movement Characteristics
and Inactive Postures

Activity/Inactivity. Subjects A, B, and C presented differing patterns of upper extremity activity: A was rather inactive during this scan, but still demonstrated abduction/adduction movements; B was continuously active, but most movements were horizontal adduction/horizontal abduction rather than abduction/adduction; C was very active, not only abducting/adducting the upper extremity, but almost continuously performing some body movements; D was different and moved from one resting posture to the next with few upper extremity movements and those occurred in only one direction. Subjects A, B, and C demonstrated a similar pattern on the Fetal Movement Time Line characterized by clusters of reversals of movement, as shown in Figure 3.

In addition, the fetal elbow was often visualized in these tapes. In subjects A, B, and C, the inactive elbow was always held at an acute angle, except when the humerus was abducted 160 degrees or more. Subject D, however, held the inactive elbow in almost full extension at all times, and spent a significant portion of the time with the head and trunk in a retroflexed posture. In fact, although referred as a low-risk pregnancy, D was described at 22 weeks as growth-retarded (a diagnosis of IUGR is not made until 25 weeks), and at 24 weeks the mother developed pregnancy-induced hypertension. Hypertension became severe enough to require hospitalization at 28 weeks, Cesarean delivery at 32 weeks, and a birth weight of three pounds, one ounce.

Velocity. Most of the abduction/adduction movements for A, B, and C were characterized by high angular velocities and large fluctuations in velocity. Some of the short-duration movements, however, had a spasmodic nature, and may be the "twitches" described in earlier studies.[5] Velocity profiles of subjects A, B and C, of the spasmodic type, were characterized by high-velocity movement in one video frame, followed by one video frame of no apparent movement, and then a comparably high velocity in the following frame. These movements occurred more frequently into adduction, but also into abduction. Subject D performed none of this type of movement.

Velocity profiles of short-duration movements contrasted with velocity profiles of the smoother type of movement (whether long or short in duration) in which there was a prolonged, gradual rise and fall in speed of movement. Many of these smoother movements can be characterized by a single video frame, partway through the movement, in which there is no apparent movement. The smooth movements do not give such a spasmodic appearance as the high-velocity pattern because the adjacent rate of movement is slower. The smoother transition in velocities yields a smoother velocity profile.

At 20 weeks of gestation, there is abundant amniotic fluid,[14] which provides resistance to fast movements. Because resistance is equal to the square of the velocity of movement,[15] any fast movements require strong muscle contraction. With weaker movements, such as observed in D, one would anticipate a paucity of movements and a lack of reversals, as was noted in the Fetal Movement Time Line. D had higher peak velocities than the others for abduction, however, although D also had less variability in peak velocities. Speed, or perhaps velocity, of fetal movement has been commented upon since Reinold[14] characterized impaired fetuses as lacking in the faster type of movements. Reinold also observed that low-risk fetuses performed both fast and slow types of movement.

Variability. Possibly, the reduced variability is a more significant feature than the actual speed. The fetus may be programmed to utilize many different velocities when moving in order to provide it with exercise under varying conditions. Perhaps, also, movement at varying velocities requires a greater degree of coordination or effort from the fetus. The small number of movements performed by D, however, limits the number of movements assessed and leaves this hypothesis quite speculative.

Glenohumeral Rhythm

deVries et al.[5] state that all movement patterns are established by 15 weeks and do not change with maturation. These investigators described movements in more global terms and did not carry out a detailed examination of the movement, as was attempted in this study. In contrast to deVries et al., Milani-Comparetti[2] believed that motor patterns are modified with maturation. Based on experience with postnatal movement, one might expect such modifications to perhaps be as subtle as changes in glenohumeral rhythm.

Results of this study suggest that not all fetuses have established the adult pattern of glenohumeral rhythm by 20 weeks. Not only is the expected ratio of one degree of scapular rotation for each two degrees of humeral movement not seen consistently, but the range of many of the scapular movements was perhaps greater than expected. Ranges of scapular elevation/depression noted in this study were sometimes 4 to 8 milliliters, which seems a considerable distance to travel on the small fetal torso.

The relatively large oscillations and ranges of motion of the scapula suggest a lack of refinement in control or a lack of stability, consistent with immaturity of movement patterns. Later in pregnancy, there is less amniotic fluid and less room, contributing to less movement and resulting in more stability. In infancy, the supine posture provides stability and the activities performed in prone serve to develop stability. Perhaps this early fetal period represents the mobility stage of motor development for the shoulder, providing extensive mobilization of the scapula in preparation for the stability tasks of infancy. There is little recorded about normal pediatric glenohumeral rhythm, but perhaps future studies will show the infant's reaching behaviors may be the beginning of controlled mobility, which would incorporate dynamic stabilization of the scapula.

Limitations

The small sample size limits the generalizability of the results. Our total subject pool consists of 12 subjects, however, and their additional data will be used to verify the preliminary results of these four subjects. Frame-by-frame analysis is extremely time-consuming but is necessary to describe subtleties of movement. Longitudinal assessment is also time-consuming but may be of extreme importance in understanding the relationship of prenatal movement to later functional behavior. In addition, the scapulohumeral angle in this study is that between the lateral border of the scapula and the humerus, rather than that used in postnatal goniometric measurement, and this provides some difficulty in determining the equivalent phase of the abduction range. Finally, the small percent of videotape in which shoulder movement occurred might suggest the need for additional imaging to determine the representative nature of the movement.

CONCLUSION

In summary, we have outlined a methodology in detail for carrying out a kinematic study of fetal movement, and presented preliminary findings regarding glenohumeral movement in the plane of the scapula. Such a study is feasible and yields reproducible findings, but is labor-intensive and usually confined to small samples. The applicability of the results to the general population will require larger studies, but the potential significance of such fetal study exists for physical and occupational therapists interested in movement characteristics of the normal and the abnormally developing child. The spatial and temporal aspects of movement are seen as a reflection of central nervous system maturation, and may form a basis for the generation of treatment strategies and progressions, especially in children with central nervous system disability.

REFERENCES

1. Marsal K. Ultrasonic assessment of fetal activity. *Clinics in Obstetrics and Gynecology.* 1983;10(3):541-563.

2. Milani-Comparetti A. The neurophysiologic and clinical implications of studies on fetal motor behaviour. *Sem Perinatol.* 1981;5:183-189.

3. Prechtl HFR. Continuity and change in early neural development. In: Prechtl HFR, ed. *Continuity of Neural Functions from Prenatal to Postnatal Life. Clinics in Developmental Medicine,*94. Oxford: Blackwell; 1984:1-15.

4. Birnholz JC, Stephens JC, Faria M. Fetal movement patterns: a possible means of defining neurologic developmental milestones in utero. *Amer J Roentgenology.* 1978;130:537-540.

5. deVries JIP, Visser GHA, Prechtl HFR. The emergence of fetal behavior. I. qualitative aspects. *Early Hum Dev.* 1982;7:17-39.

6. Ianniruberto A, Tajani E. Ultrasonographic study of fetal movements. Ultrasonic study of fetal movements. *Sem Perinatol.* 1981;5:175-181.

7. deVries JIP, Visser GHA, Prechtl HFR. The emergence of fetal behavior. II.quantitative aspects. *Early Hum Dev.* 1985;12:41-63.

8. O'Rahilly R, Gardner E. The timing and sequence of events in the development of the limbs in the human embryo. *Anat Embryol.* 1975;1:148.

9. Lewis WH. The development of the arm in man. *Am J Anat.* 1902; 1(2):145-184.

10. Hooker D. *The Prenatal Origin of Behavior.* Lawrence, KA: University of Kansas Press; 1952.

11. Gardner E, Gray DJ. Prenatal development of the human shoulder and acromioclavicular joints. *Am J Anat.* 1953;92:219-276.

12. Hardy MA, Macdonald JA, Kuder S. *The ABC: Assessment of Behavioral Components*. Springfield, IL: Charles C. Thomas; 1988.

13. Norkin CC and Levangie PK. *Joint Structure and Function. A Comprehensive Analysis*. Philadelphia, FA Davis, 1992.

14. Reinold E. Clinical value of fetal spontaneous movements in early pregnancy. *J Perinatol Med.* 1973;1:65-69.

15. Hall S. *Basic Biomechanics*. St. Louis, MI: Mosby Year Book Inc.;1991.

The Development of Fetal Behaviors
and Their Relationship
to Neonatal Behavioral Organization

Ann Marie MacLeod
Joyce W. Sparling

SUMMARY. Neonatal behaviors described by Als were observed in the fetus, and the relationship of these fetal motor behaviors to neonatal behavioral organization was investigated. A convenience sample of three low-risk women and their fetuses was identified early in pregnancy and followed through birth. Ultrasound imagings of these fetuses were videotaped at 12, 14, and 16 weeks of gestation, and the Assessment of Preterm Infant Behaviors (APIB) was administered at 42 weeks corrected age. Of the 20 neonatal behaviors described by Als and selected for coding in the fetus, 80% were observed at 12 weeks, 70% at 14 weeks, and 40% at 16 weeks of gestation. At 16 weeks, 87-99 percent of the behaviors scored were those considered regulatory by Als and therefore suggestive of some fetal behavioral organization at this gestational age for these subjects. No apparent relationship existed between early fetal movement in terms of the frequency and duration of the behaviors described by Als and neonatal behavioral organization as measured by the APIB. Results suggest that the neonatal behaviors described by Als can be used to de-

Ann Marie MacLeod completed her advanced graduate degree in physical therapy at the University of North Carolina at Chapel Hill and is now affiliated with an international research organization based in Colorado. Joyce W. Sparling, PhD, PT, OT, is Assistant Professor in the Division of Physical Therapy at the University of North Carolina at Chapel Hill. She is Project Director for the Maternal and Child Health Postgraduate Training Grant.

This study was completed as partial fulfillment for the Master of Science degree in physical therapy at the University of North Carolina at Chapel Hill. The study was supported in part by the Maternal and Child Health Grant 149 from the Department of Health and Human Services and by the Pediatric Teaching Unit, Wake Area Health Education Center, Raleigh, North Carolina.

scribe fetal movement, but their frequency and duration may not be a sufficient measure of fetal organization.

Prechtl,[1] Milani Comparetti[2] and others have suggested that functional relationships exist between fetal and neonatal behaviors. The continuity of competence from the fetal to neonatal period is a question of some importance that might lead to the identification of levels of behavioral organization in the young fetus. Continuity of competence of newborn and older infants has been addressed by Als,[3] who has identified a number of motor behaviors to assist in the study of continuity of competence and behavioral organization over time. These behaviors may also be able to be used to describe fetal behavior. To address the continuum of motor behaviors across the birth transition, these functional motor descriptors were used in a pilot study of fetal and neonatal movement. The purposes of this exploratory study were to investigate the development of fetal motor behaviors according to the neonatal assessment described by Als, to study the relationship between fetal and neonatal behaviors, and to describe the use of these behaviors in evaluating behavioral organization.

BEHAVIORAL ORGANIZATION

Behavioral organization is the ability to maintain or regain stable autonomic functioning, to modulate motor behaviors, to access a wide range of states, and to control responses to external and internal stimulation.[3] Current theories[3,4] suggest that the movement of the fetus may play a significant role in postnatal behavioral organization and the development of motor coordination.

Synactive Theory

The Synactive Theory[3] is a process-oriented model used to understand the behavioral development and organization of individual neonates. This theory focuses on the dynamic, continuous interplay of five subsystems of the organism, and the organism's continuous transactions with the environment. The subsystems are the autonomic, motor, state, attention-interaction, and self-regulatory subsystems. The *autonomic* subsystem output can be observed in the patterns of respiration, color change, tremulousness and visceral signs such as gagging and hiccoughing. The *motor* subsystem is observable in the balance and control of posture, tone, and movement. The *state* subsystem involves the range of states available from sleeping to aroused, the clarity of the states, and the pattern of transition from one state to another. The *attention-interaction* subsystem is observed in the ability to come to a quiet alert state and to utilize the state to take in cognitive and social-emotional information from the environment. The *self-regulatory* system is observed in an infant's strategies to maintain and regain behavioral organization.

In the Synactive Theory, functional organization is interpreted in part in terms of dual antagonistic behaviors. The principle of dual antagonist integration suggests that an organism exhibits two basic kinds of opposing responses and strives for integration of these responses.[5] While striving for integration, tension within an organism is created between these exploratory and withdrawing responses. If the input and the internal readiness of the organism are matched, the organism will explore the input, and will react and interact with it. As the input reaches the organism's internal tolerance threshold, withdrawal responses may be released simultaneously with the exploratory responses. When the tolerance threshold is exceeded, the exploratory responses may abruptly switch to withdrawal responses.

Using the principles of dual antagonist integration, Als classified neonatal motor behaviors as either approach/self-regulation or avoidance/stress behaviors. Approach/self-regulatory behaviors are strategies an infant uses to explore self and the environment and to maintain or regain behavioral organization. As a general rule, approach behaviors are movements into flexion and are more variable and differentiated than avoidance behaviors. Avoidance/stress behaviors are strategies or behaviors which infants use to move away from or protect themselves from a potential threat, or behaviors used to avoid environmental demands that are inappropriate for the infant either in complexity, intensity, or timing. As a general rule, avoidance behaviors are movements into extension and are more global in their expression than regulatory behaviors.

Als[3] suggests that approach/withdrawal behaviors have meaning and are functional in that they provide channels for infant communication. Using a dual antagonistic system, infants are able to communicate to a caretaker when they are generally organized or disorganized, when a stimulus is within or beyond their tolerance threshold, and when they need assistance. Whether this interpretation is applicable to the fetus is unknown, but the behaviors themselves may be able to be observed in the fetus and may suggest a continuity of competence across the birth transition.

Dynamic Pattern Theory

The Synactive Theory is consistent with ideas fundamental to the dynamic systems theory and dynamic pattern theory. Together these theories provide a unique understanding of behavioral changes and subsystem influences. One fundamental assumption of dynamic theory is that developing organisms are complex, cooperative systems that interact with one another. All systems must participate in a cooperative way to insure a functionally appropriate outcome.[6]

A second assumption of dynamic systems theory is that the system exists within a specific context that must be recognized as a major determinant of the system's functional performance. As in the Synactive Theory, the infant does not move in an environmental vacuum but is in continuous transaction with the environment. Sameroff and Chandler's[7] transactional model stresses the importance of an ongoing, reciprocal relationship between the child and the caregiving environment. Neither the child nor the caregiving environment is constant but change as a function of mutual influences. The environment in which the child develops can either enhance or detract from that child's developmental potential.[8]

The third fundamental assumption of dynamic systems is that a developing system has certain self-organizing properties. Self-organization is the ability to form patterns spontaneously from the interaction of the component parts.[6] This view of self-organization is mirrored in one of the basic concepts of Als, that of the transformation of skills.[9] This concept states that skills and functions may be explained in terms of spontaneous formation of new patterns. The process of transformation depends upon the continuous interaction of subsystems or component parts. Although Als supports the hypothesis of transformation of functions, she also believes that a continuity of competence or a consistency is evident in the way in which individuals interact with their environment over their life span.[9]

Continuity of Competency

Continuity of competency also refers to an individual consistency in the underlying organizational patterns of form and function.[10] The task, function, or skill may be transformed or changed with development, but the fundamental form of the interaction is the same.[11] An infant's means of mobility may change from crawling to walking, but the underlying quality of movement is consistent, a concept not always synchronous with therapeutic hypotheses.

To assess the continuity of an individual's neurobehavioral competency, Als designed two scales. The Assessment of Preterm Infants' Behavior (APIB)[12] was developed for use in the newborn period, while the Kangaroo-Box Paradigm,[13] a play situation, was designed for use at older ages. The APIB was given to 160 healthy preterm and full term infants at 42 weeks of gestation and the Kangaroo-Box was given to these same children at nine months of age. Cluster analysis at each age yielded three behaviorally distinct groups of infants. Cluster one infants were the most competent or organized, while cluster three infants were the least competent or most disorganized infants. Consistency of cluster membership from the newborn period to nine months was significant, supporting the hypothesis that neurobehavioral competence is consistent across time.[9]

In a subsequent study[14] of 98 healthy preterm and full term infants, the APIB was robust in assessing neurobehavioral competency, independent of an infant's gestational age at birth. Of the 98 infants, 34 were full term infants. Full term infants were found in each of the three clusters, demonstrating that even full term infants vary in neurobehavioral competencies and that the APIB is a sensitive measure of those differences. The child's neurobehavioral competencies may be expressed by the effectiveness of an infant's self-regulatory or approach strategies, but this perspective has not been described in relation to the fetus.

Support exists, however, for the continuity of competent behaviors from intrauterine to extrauterine environment. Prechtl[1,p8] states, "While birth is an environmental discontinuity par excellence, the neurological repertoire displays an impressive continuity around the transition from intrauterine to extrauterine life." The concept of continuity of behaviors was further supported by a study of preterm infants[15] in which preterm infants did not change their motor repertoire at birth around 40 weeks of gestation. In addition, Milani Comparetti[2] concluded that the fetus has the full repertoire of movements and, therefore, no movement patterns originate at birth. Further support for this perspective is found in Robertson's[16] investigation of cyclic motility. Cyclic patterns of spontaneous movement remained unchanged during active sleep from the fetal to the neonatal period. Based on this support for continuity of competence, a preliminary descriptive study was designed to observe early fetal motor behaviors and investigate their relationship to neonatal behavioral competence. If competency is consistent across time, assessment of fetal movement may provide a tool for the early determination of neurobehavioral competency and lead to early assessment and even intervention, when warranted.

METHOD

Subjects

This study was conducted as part of a multidimensional study of fetal movement.[17] A convenience sample of three women was selected from a private obstetric practice at a tertiary-care hospital. At the time of identification, the women were less than 12 weeks pregnant, had a single pregnancy, and were described as having a low-risk pregnancy (North Carolina Memorial Hospital Fetal Risk Form). These women were Caucasian, from 26 to 30 years of age, and were health care professionals. Two of the three fetuses were born prematurely: subject 4 at 35 weeks gestational age (GA) and subject 6 at 37 weeks GA. No known etiology for either premature delivery was determined. Subject 5 was born at 40 weeks of gestation. All of the newborn infants were average weight for their gestational age: two were male and one was female. Maternal subjects gave informed consent in which they agreed to three, 30-minute ultrasound (US) imagings during pregnancy and to an APIB[18] at their infant's corrected age of 42 weeks. That age was selected in order to ensure physiological stability of the neonates and permit comparison across subjects.

Instrumentation

Ultrasound imagings were recorded using a 3.5 mHz linear array transducer. A player/recorder and a high-resolution monitor were used for replaying the videotapes of these imagings for scoring.

The Assessment of Preterm Infant Behavior (APIB)[18] is an extension of the Brazelton Neonatal Behavioral Assessment Scale.[19] The numerous items of the APIB are arranged into a graded sequence of six increasingly demanding "packages" of stimulation. The assessment starts with distal stimulation that is presented during sleep, moves to tactile and vestibular stimulation, and finally to auditory and visual stimulation. During the assessment, the examiner monitors the infant's behaviors along six subsystems: autonomic, motor, state, attention/interaction, self-regulation, and the infant's response to examiner facilitation. The six subsystem summary scores are considered to be key parameters of the APIB.

After observation and scoring of specific behaviors, the APIB can be reduced to 32 a priori summary variables,[20] of which eight were used in this study: the six subsystem summary scores, plus the motor system regulatory score and the motor system stress score. The regulatory and stress scores were chosen because they are summaries of motor performance. Subsystem summary scores range from 1 to 9 with "1" representing the optimal and "9" the poorest performance. Motor system regulatory and stress scores range from zero to three with "0" indicating the behavior was not observed, and a score of "3" indicating the behavior was frequently observed.

The stress and regulatory behaviors are defined in the Manual for the Naturalistic Observation of Newborn Behavior,[18] and a brief description of them is given in Table 1. Motor behaviors that are described by Als, but are not included in the study were grimace,

TABLE 1.   Self-Regulatory/Approach and Stress/Withdrawal
Behaviors of the Assessment of Preterm Infant Behavior(APIB)

REGULATORY BEHAVIORS

Grasp	Opening and closing of the hands.
Hand clasp	Hands come in contact with each other either holding, pressing against, or interdigitating.
Hand on face	Hands placed palm up or down on facial area.
Hand to mouth	Attempted or successful hand/fingers to mouth.
Foot clasp	Sole of foot positioned against other sole or leg, or legs crossed,usually at ankles.
Holding on	A successful grasp for a duration.
Leg brace	Lower limb extension to uterine wall.
Sucking	Rhythmical opening and closing of mouth.
Suck search	Mouth opening in a searching mode.
Tuck Trunk	Trunk movement into flexion: can include leg flexion.

STRESS BEHAVIORS

Airplane	Shoulder abduction.
Arch	Trunk and head extension.
Diffuse squirm	Small wiggling movements of trunk
Finger splay	Fingers extend and abduct.
Fisting	Finger flexion into a fist.
Gape face	Mouth droop.
Mouthing	More than one opening and closing of mouth.
Salute	Arm extension.
Sitting-on-air	Hips flexed and knees extended.
Stretch/drown	"Labored" trunk extension followed by trunk flexion attempts.

tongue extension, and smiling, soft tissue movements that are difficult to detect on US image. The APIB is used only by certified APIB examiners who have achieved 90%-95% interrater reliability with an APIB trainer.

Procedure

Pilot Study. A pilot study was conducted to determine if approach and avoidance behaviors were observable in the young fetus, and if present, could be reliably scored. Thirty-minute US imagings of three fetuses were selected from our bank of fetal imaging tapes[17] and were coded by the first author to determine the frequency of approach and avoidance behaviors at 14 and 16 weeks of gestation. Eighty-five percent of motor behaviors described by Als were observed. Ten percent of the US imagings were then randomly selected to be coded by an obstetrician experienced in assessing diagnostic US imagings and a person certified as an APIB tester. The obstetrician's descriptions were compared with coded tapes and 100 percent agreement on occurrence of specific behaviors was reached in the first viewing. The APIB tester was not accustomed to observing US images, but after an hour-long training session obtained 90 percent agreement with the first author.

Main Study. Ultrasound imagings were conducted between 4 and 6 PM in a quiet room by a certified ultrasonographer with the pregnant woman in a semi-recumbent position. In the initial two minutes of imaging, the US technician oriented the maternal subject to fetal body parts. To determine the gestational age of the fetus, crown/rump measurements were taken at 12 weeks, and femoral length and biparietal diameter measurements were taken at 14 and 16 weeks. After the subject was oriented and measurements recorded, 30 minutes of US imagings were recorded by an assistant in order to insure unbiased coding of the fetal movements and of the APIB testing.

An APIB was conducted in the home at 42 weeks corrected age by the first author who was unaware of the performance of the child as a fetus. To maximize opportunity for observing neonatal alertness and orientation, the APIB was conducted midway between feedings and took an average of 45 minutes to complete.

The videotaped imagings of the fetus were later coded for frequency and duration of the 20 individual approach and avoidance behaviors described in Table 1. At the time of coding, a time code of minutes, seconds, and hundredths of a second was burned onto a second-generation videotape. Each US imaging was viewed three times: once to code upper extremity and facial behaviors, once to code the lower extremities and tuck trunk, and the third time to code trunk behaviors other than tuck trunk. Each 30 minutes of US imaging required 4.5 to 6.5 hours for coding. The first author assessed the subjects with the APIB prior to assessing the videotapes of the US imagings. She was blinded to subject identity when coding the US imagings.

Analysis

Scoreable portions of US imagings were identified and the percent of tape usable for analysis was calculated. Unscoreable time included time when the picture of the fetus was out of focus and time when movements other than those motor behaviors described by Als were observed. The number, frequency, and duration of approach and avoidance behaviors observed at 12, 14, and 16 weeks GA was recorded.

To control for different activity levels among fetuses, the ratios of avoidance/total behaviors and approach/total behaviors were calculated for both the frequency and duration. The trends in frequency and duration ratios from 12 to 14 to 16 weeks GA were described. To investigate the relationship between these fetal motor behaviors and neonatal behavioral organization, frequency and duration ratios of the fetal behaviors were descriptively compared to eight neonatal a priori summary scores on the APIB.

RESULTS

Scoreable portions of the 30-minute US imagings varied somewhat across the different gestational ages and across the subjects. The mean amount of usable tape at 12 weeks GA was 14 minutes, 27 seconds and 55 frames; at 14 weeks was 16 minutes, 57 seconds and 61 frames; and for 16 weeks was 13 minutes, 59 seconds and 70 frames. The mean amount of usable tape for subject 4 was 15 minutes, 31 seconds and 78 frames; for subject 5 was 14 minutes, 42 seconds and 64 frames; and for subject 6 was 14 minutes, 51 seconds and 61 frames.

Motor Behaviors Observed

Sixteen of the 20 neonatal motor behaviors described by Als[3] were observed in the 12-16 week low-risk fetus. Three behaviors considered by Als to be stress-related, and one behavior considered to be self-regulatory were not observed.

The percent of avoidance and approach behaviors observed decreased from 12 to 14 to 16 weeks GA. Approach behaviors had a 43 percent reduction (9 to 8 to 6 behaviors), while avoidance behaviors had a 71 percent reduction (7 to 6 to 2 behaviors). Eighty percent of the 20 motor behaviors coded were observed at 12 weeks GA (9/10 approach and 7/10 avoidance behaviors). Motor behaviors not observed were airplane, fisting, gape face, and sucking. Seventy percent of the 20 motor behaviors were observed at 14 weeks GA (8/10 approach behaviors, 6/10 avoidance behaviors). Those not observed were airplane, fisting, gape face, holding on, stretch/drown, and sucking. Forty percent of identified behaviors were observed at 16 weeks GA (6/10 approach and 2/10 avoidance behaviors). Motor behaviors not observed were airplane, arch, diffuse squirm, fisting, gape face, holding on, salute, sitting on air, stretch/drown, sucking, suck search, and tuck.

The frequency of those motor behaviors observed increased from 12 to 14 weeks and decreased from 14 to 16 weeks in two fetuses. The overall activity level in the third fetus remained the same from 12 to 14 weeks and decreased from 14 to 16 weeks.

Frequency Ratio

The mean frequency ratio of approach/total motor behaviors increased from 12 to 16 weeks, while the mean frequency ratio of avoidance/total motor behaviors decreased, as shown in Figure 1. The mean frequency ratio of approach/total behaviors at 16 weeks

FIGURE 1. Mean Frequency of Approach and Avoidance Behaviors at Three Gestational Ages

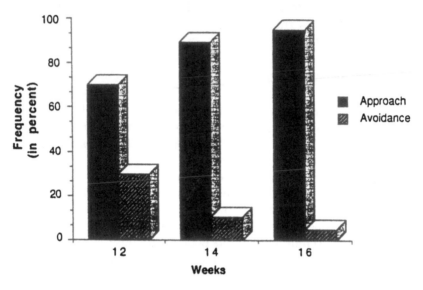

was 95 percent. The mean frequency ratio of avoidance/total behaviors at 16 weeks was 5 percent.

The increase from 12 to 14 weeks of gestation was noted in all three fetuses, as shown in Figure 2. From 14 to 16 weeks of gestation, the frequency ratio of approach/total motor behaviors increased in two fetuses and slightly decreased in the third. The percent frequency of avoidance/total motor behaviors showed the opposite trends, decreasing from 12 to 16 weeks, as shown in Figure 3. The decrease from 12 to 14 weeks occurred in all three fetuses. From 14 to 16 weeks, the avoidance/total behaviors continued to decrease in two fetuses, and slightly increased in the third fetus.

Duration

The mean percent durations of the 16 motor behaviors showed the same trend as the frequency ratios. The mean percent duration of approach/total behaviors increased from 12 to 16 weeks, while the mean percent duration of avoidance/total behaviors decreased

FIGURE 2. Frequency of Approach Behaviors for Three Fetuses at Three Gestational Ages

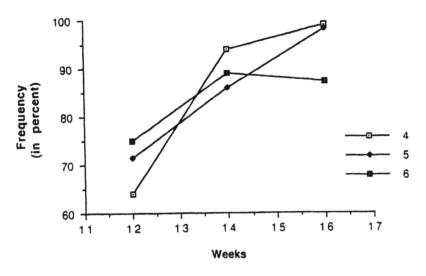

FIGURE 3. Frequency of Avoidance Behaviors for Three Subjects at Three Gestational Ages

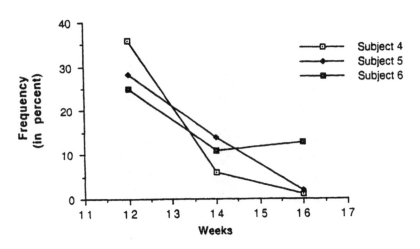

during this time span, as shown in Figure 4. At 16 weeks, the mean duration ratio of approach/total behaviors was 99 percent, while the mean duration ratio of avoidance/total behaviors was 1 percent.

For two of the three fetuses (subjects 4 and 6), the duration ratio of approach/total motor behaviors increased minimally from 12 to 14 to 16 weeks. For a third fetus (subject 5), the ratio decreased from 12 to 14 weeks but increased from 14 to 16 weeks. Avoidance/total motor behaviors in two of the three fetuses decreased minimally from 12 to 14 to 16 weeks GA. The third fetus increased from 12 to 14 weeks but decreased from 14 to 16 weeks.

Neonatal Scores

The six summary, and the regulatory and stress scores on the APIB are shown in Table 2. The neonate born at 35 weeks had the least favorable motor summary score of 4.17, the highest regulatory score and a low stress score; the neonate born at 37 weeks had the mid-range motor summary score of 3.67 and mid-range regulatory and stress scores; the full term neonate had the best motor summary

FIGURE 4. Mean Duration of Approach and Avoidance Behaviors at Three Gestational Ages

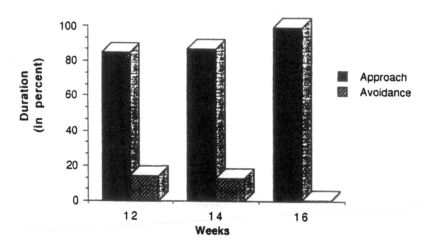

TABLE 2.   Subsystem Summary Scores from the Assessment of
Preterm Infant Behaviors

APIB Summary Scores	Subjects		
	4	5	6
	Preterm 35 weeks	Fullterm 40 weeks	Preterm 37 weeks
*Autonomic	4.06	3.27	4.83
*Motor	4.17	2.44	3.67
*State	5.00	3.33	4.06
*Attention/Interaction	5.33	6.00	5.33
*Self-Regulation	5.89	5.61	4.89
*Facilitation	6.17	5.50	6.17
**Motor Regulatory Score	1.91	1.17	1.33
**Motor Stress Score	.67	.11	.33

*A score of one represents the optimal performance and nine the
poorest

**A score of zero indicates the behaviors were not observed and
score of three indicates the behaviors were frequently observed

score of 2.44, a mid-range regulatory score and a low stress score.
Other scores were in the middle performance range.

A relationship between regulatory and stress summary scores
appeared to exist. Subjects who had the highest (1.91), mid (1.33),
or lowest (1.17) score on the regulatory score also had the highest
(.67), mid (.33), or lowest (.11) score on the avoidance score.

Relationship Between Fetal and Neonatal Scores

Little variance was observed across the scores for fetuses and
neonates, as shown in Figures 2 and 3 and in Table 2. The three
subjects appeared to perform within similar ranges for frequency
and duration of motor behaviors early in pregnancy and for neonatal APIB Summary scores.

DISCUSSION

Most of the neonatal behaviors described by Als were observed in the young fetus. More of the behaviors termed regulatory or approach were observed than the behaviors termed stress or avoidance, and more of these regulatory behaviors were noted at 16 weeks than at 12 weeks. That a complete repertoire of motor patterns is available to the low-risk young fetus is consistent with other studies. Seven of the nine movement patterns identified by Birnholz[21] were observed by 15 weeks with the isolated diaphragm and respiratory movements occurring after 20 weeks. The 16 behaviors Ianniruberto and Tajani[22] identified were all observed by 20 weeks of gestation, while the 16 movements identified by deVries, Visser and Prechtl[23] were all observed by 15 weeks.

Results from this study provide some evidence for development of fetal behaviors proceeding from a global state to one of increasing differentiation.[3,24] Avoidance behaviors have been described as more global behaviors, while approach behaviors are more variable and differentiated. The observed reduction of avoidance behaviors over time and the proportional increase of approach behaviors suggests some support for this perspective and an increasing organization of the fetus from 12 to 16 weeks of gestation.

No apparent relationship was found between fetal motor behavior and neonatal behavioral organization to support the concept of continuity of competency. One possible explanation is that the fetus and neonate were evaluated in different contexts.[4] Neonates were taken through a series of manipulations and hence given the opportunity to reach their threshold of behavioral organization, while fetuses were observed in their natural environment without manipulation. Unlike the neonates, the fetuses' behavioral organization was not able to be observed through a range of environmental challenges. This suggests that permissive conditions are critical to the expression of motor behaviors, a central concept to dynamic systems theory.

Another factor which affects our ability to test continuity of competency from the fetus to the neonate is the operational definition of fetal organization. Frequency and duration of approach and avoidance behaviors did not appear to be sensitive measures of fetal motor organization. Future studies will need to focus on developing a qualitative fetal motor scale taking into consideration approach and avoidance behaviors, as described in this issue by Green and Sparling.

In order to study fetal organization, fetal behaviors were grouped into discrete categories of approach or avoidance behaviors. An arm extension (avoidance), for example, was part of a series of movements that ended with the hand at the mouth (approach). Future studies may more appropriately consider movement in context rather than grouping behaviors into a priori dual antagonistic categories.

In addition, other variables may be used to assess fetal motor organization. For example, state variables can be used to assess the more mature fetus.[25] To identify variables that may be related to fetal motor organization, a study comparing fetal movement of high-risk and low-risk pregnancies is being planned by Sparling and Katz. The high risk pregnancy may provide an environment that challenges fetal motor organization beyond the threshold of organization.

Prematurity may have acted as a confounding variable in determining the relationship between fetal motor behaviors and neonatal behavioral organization. Prematurity appeared to be related to the motor subsystem summary score as shown in Table 2. The full term infant had the best motor summary score followed by the infant born at 37 weeks, and then the infant born at 35 weeks. These scores could be a reflection of problems associated with prematurity, as premature neonates have been scored on the APIB as having less well organized motor subsystems than full term neonates.[13]

In a cluster analysis of APIB scores on 98 full term and preterm infants, the well organized group had a mean score of 2.37 which was significantly different from the less well organized group with a mean score of 3.28.[14] A motor summary score of 2.44 (subject 5) may represent a significantly more organized motor summary score than 3.67 (subject 6) or 4.17 (subject 4).

One possible explanation for the apparent relationship between motor regulatory scores and motor stress scores is that infants who have a less organized motor subsystem need to make more attempts to regulate their motor system. For example, the subject born at 35 weeks (subject 4) was the least organized on the motor subsystem summary variable, and had the highest stress score, and the highest motor regulatory score. Conversely, the full term neonate (subject 5) had the lowest scores on regulatory and motor scores, and was the most motorically organized, suggesting fewer efforts were needed to regulate his motor subsystem.

Limitations

Limitations included the small sample size, the possible confound of prematurity, and the percent of ultrasound imagings that were unscoreable. The scoring of fetal movement is labor-intensive, limiting the number of subjects whose movements can be precisely scored. More subjects would have included a greater number of full term births for comparison. Even though APIB testing was conducted at 42 weeks corrected age, performance of the two premature subjects could have affected the results. The high percentage of imagings that were unscoreable either because of the view or of transducer movement, or because behaviors other than the behaviors described by Als were seen, was somewhat consistent across the sample.

Whether the behaviors noted for these three subjects were typical is not known. It was surprising that sucking and suck search were not observed, since those are commonly observed behaviors among other investigators and within our own data pool. In addition to those behaviors described by Als, other movements frequently observed in the fetus were hands to the knees or feet, and hand behind the head. These behaviors were not considered in this study, but may be important indicators of fetal organization.

This study did not differentiate among the various expressions of a behavior, for instance, hand to mouth has a variety of expressions; hand near the mouth, hand to the mouth, both hands to the mouth, hand to the mouth with hand clasp, hand to the mouth with mouthing, hand to mouth maintained in position vs. a sequence of repeated hand to mouth movements. The development of a variety of expressions of a fetal behavior may be an important facet of fetal movement and development.

CONCLUSION AND IMPLICATIONS

The study demonstrates that the behaviors described by Als can be observed in the young fetus. Their use may augment existing assessments of fetal movement and further support the measurement of fetal and neonatal movement and the issue of continuity of competence. Future fetal assessment, however, may need to include more than the motor subsystem in order to validly measure neurobehavioral competency.

Results suggest that neural circuitry and permissive environmental conditions must be present in order for behaviors to be expressed.[26] Nine of ten approach behaviors were present at 12 weeks gestational age suggesting that the neural circuitry and permissive conditions for the expression of these behaviors were present at that time. This finding has implications when considering the premature infant in the neonatal intensive care unit. The infant in this unnatural environment is essentially a "displaced fetus."[10] If the neural circuitry is present for motor approach behaviors at 12 weeks of gestation, and if 99 percent of the dual antagonistic behaviors observed in the 16-week fetus are approach behaviors, then a goal in a neonatal intensive care unit would be to provide conditions that permit a high proportion of the neonate's behaviors to be approach behaviors. Gravity may be providing an initial insurmountable challenge to the preterm.

Premature infants are often rated as more irritable and less able to maintain quiet states than full term infants.[27] This difference may be partially due to a lack of practice of approach or self-regulatory behaviors that may be the result of an unsupportive extrauterine environment. Providing a supportive environment is a continuous challenge for NICU caregivers.[10]

REFERENCES

1. Prechtl HFR. *Continuity and change in early neural development. Clinics in Developmental Medicine.* Philadelphia, NJ: JB Lippincott; 1984.

2. Milani Comparetti A. Pattern analysis of normal and abnormal development: the fetus, the newborn, the child, In: Slaton DS, ed. *Development of Movement in Infancy.* Chapel Hill, NC; 1981:1-37.

3. Als H. Toward a synactive theory in development: promise for the assessment and support of infant individuality. *Infant Mental Health Journal.* 1982;3(4): 229-243.

4. Thelen E, Ulrich BD. *Hidden Skills.* Monographs of the Society for Research in Child Development, Serial #223. 1991;56(1).

5. Denny-Brown D. *The Cerebral Control of Movement*. Springfield, IL: Charles C. Thomas;1966.

6. Thelen E, Ulrich BD, Jensen JL. The developmental origins of locomotion. In: Woollacott M, Shumway-Cook A, eds. *The Development of Posture and Gait Across the Lifespan*. Columbia, SC: University of South Carolina Press; 1989:25-47.

7. Sameroff AJ, Chandler MJ. Reproductive risk and the continuum of care-taking casualty. In: Horowitz FD, Hetherington M, Scarr-Salapatek S, Siegel G, eds. *Review of Child Development Research*. 1975;4:187-244. Chicago, IL: University of Chicago.

8. O'Donnell K. The family system in neonatal care: theoretical perspectives, In: Slaton D, ed. *Advances in Neonatal Special Care*. Chapel Hill, NC;1985:107-115.

9. Als H, Duffy F, McAnulty GB. Neurobehavioral competence in healthy preterm and fullterm infants: newborn period to 9 months. *Dev Pediatr*, in press.

10. Als H. Self-regulation and motor development in preterm infants. In: Lockman J, Hazen N, eds. *Action in Social Context. Perspectives on Early Development*. New York, NY: Plenum;1989:65-97.

11. Knobloch H, Pasamanick B. Prediction from the assessment of neuromotor and intellectual status in infancy, In: Zubin J, Jervis GA, eds. *Psychopathology of Mental Development*. New York, NY: Grune and Stratton;1967:81-87.

12. Als H, Lester BM, Tronick EZ, Brazelton TB. Manual for the Assessment of Preterm Infants' Behavior (APIB). In: Fitzgerald H, Lester BM, Yogman MW, eds. *Theory and Research in Behavioral Pediatrics*. New York, NY: Plenum. 1982;1:65-132.

13. Als H, Duffy F, McAnulty GB. Behavioral differences between preterm and full-term newborns as measured with the APIB system scores:I. *Inf Behav Dev*. 1988;11:305-318.

14. Als H, Duffy F, McAnulty GB. The APIB, an assessment of functional competence in preterm and fullterm newborns regardless of gestational age at birth:II. *Inf Behav Dev*. 1988;11:319-331.

15. Prechtl HFR, Fargel JW, Weinmann HM, Bakker HH. Posture, motility and respiration of low-risk pre-term infants. *Dev Med Child Neurol*. 1979;21:3-27.

16. Robertson SS. Human cyclic motility: fetal-newborn continuities and newborn state differences. *Dev Psychobiol*. 1987;20(4):425-442.

17. Sparling JW, Wilhelm IJ, MacLeod AM, Greene S, Katz V, Blanchard G, Huntington G. Developing a taxonomy of fetal movement: the first step in a longitudinal collaborative study. *Phys Occup Ther Pediatr*. 1990;10(1):43-46.

18. Als H. Manual for the naturalistic observation of newborn behavior (preterm and fullterm infants). Available from author. 1984.

19. Brazelton TB. The neonatal behavioral assessment scale. *Clinics in Developmental Medicine* (2nd ed.). Philadelphia, PA: Lippincott;1984.

20. Als H. APIB features:summary variables. Available from author, 1987.

21. Birnholz JC, Stephens JC, Faria M. Fetal movement patterns: a possible means of defining neurologic developmental milestones in utero. *Am J Roentgenol*. 1978;130:537-540.

22. Ianniruberto A, Tajani E. Ultrasonographic study of fetal movements. *Semin Perinatol.* 1981;5(2):175-181.

23. de Vries JIP, Visser GHA, Prechtl HFR. The emergence of fetal behaviour, 1. Qualitative aspects. *Early Hum Dev.* 1982;7:301-322.

24. Dabrowksi K. Peichowski MM. *Theory of Levels of Emotional Development: Multilevelness and Positive Disintegration.* Oceanside, NY:Dabor Science Publications;1977.

25. Hume RF Jr, O'Donnell KJ, Stanger CL, Killam AP, Gingras JL. In utero cocaine exposure: observations of fetal behavioral state may predict neonatal outcome. *Amer J Obstet Gynecol.* 1989;161:685-690.

26. Bekoff A, Kauer JA. Neural control of hatching: fate of the pattern generator for the leg movements of hatching in posthatching chicks. *J Neurosci.* 1984;4: 2659-2666.

27. McGehee LJ, Eckerman CO. The preterm infant as a social partner: responsive but unreadable. *Inf Behav Dev.* 1983;6:461-470.

The Future of Fetal Imaging: One Person's Perspective

E.A. Lyons

It is easy to write about the future while flying at 35,000 feet. In fact, this is an ideal locale for the "blue sky" approach to looking towards the future of fetal imaging.

As a radiologist trained in ultrasound imaging with a special interest in the developing fetus, this is a unique opportunity to step back from a view that stresses *morphology*, to explore the bounds as they are being described by the physiotherapy community. To deal on a day-to-day basis with the end result of a nine-month period of growth and development, the physiotherapist must assess patterns of motion in the newborn child and, from a knowledge base of normal, deal with the abnormal.

But–when did it all start? How early in development is motion detectable in utero? What are the normal patterns and can one identify those patterns that deviate from the norm early enough to intervene? Can one understand why the deviation occurs and if it is possible to correct it? How will developments in computer technology affect the changes in the ultrasound scanners of tomorrow? For how much longer will we be bound by the technological chains of today?

Fetal motion studies are really in their infancy–not because of a lack of scientific curiosity–but, I believe, because of a lack of adequate technology. Relative to what will be available in five years, we are in the *ultrasonic stone age*. The images that we can craft are

E.A. Lyons, FRCP(C), FACR, MD, is Professor of Radiology and Obstetrics & Gynecology, Associate Professor of Anatomy, and Chairman of the Department of Radiology, University of Manitoba.

227

limited in time and space. Single *"slices"* of the fetus viewed during brief periods of limited activity can create in the minds' eye of the sonic observer a pseudo three-dimensional image. "Pseudo" in that it is only as good as the trained *inner eye* of the observer. It is highly dependent on the complexity of the object scanned and can only be viewed by the observer and, at that, only for as long as the activity of this inner vision is retained. These reflect the flaws of the present and present the challenges for the future.

WHAT CAN WE DO TODAY–IN 1992?

We use real time imaging to view "slices" or "planes" of an object, ergo–"planar imaging." A single row of more than 100 ultrasound crystals generate an ultrasound beam 10-15 cm wide that can give "high" resolution slices. High resolution means being able to differentiate two objects 1-2 mms apart. This beam can encompass the entire, early embryo but only a part of the fetus in the second and third trimesters. Image resolution improves with higher frequency transducers (5 to 10 Mhz) and is further improved by using broad band crystals that enable engineers to utilize the highest frequency sound for structures close to the transducer and the lower frequency sound for those deeper in the body. This "simple" manoeuvre of creating *variable frequency transducers* has overcome one of the major compromises of the past twenty years–the single frequency transducer. With a fixed frequency probe one could clearly focus on only one area at a time. The early attempts to overcome this incorporated two or more fixed frequency crystals into a single transducer, thus allowing the operator some flexibility. This approach was totally inadequate with the introduction of color Doppler and the birth of three-dimensional ultrasound. These were crude beginnings when viewed in the scope of what is now possible and what should be possible in the future.

Color Doppler imaging is now the standard for the examination of many organ systems and in the "near" future, three to five years from now, will be THE standard for all organ systems. The rate-limiting factor today is the cost, but as the whole system is reduced to a single computer chip, the costs will drop substantially. I predict that we will be able to purchase a color Doppler scanner for $50,000 to $75,000 within the next three to five years. Systems are now readily available with high sensitivity to detect very low rates of blood flow (down to 0.3 cm/sec) and small volumes of flow in very small vessels. But to what end? In obstetrics today we use color Doppler imaging to measure flow velocity in fetal umbilical vessels, the fetal aorta and carotid arteries. Evidence of low diastolic flow indicates a high resistance which may be associated with intrauterine growth retardation. Work has focused on developing ratios of flow velocity using a variety of different vessels. The most frequently used indices are the pulsatility and resistive indices of the umbilical artery alone or in comparison with fetal aortic or carotid flow. Although these findings show great promise, the technique is still not widely used.

Endocavitary ultrasound has added a new dimension to imaging the embryo and fetus. Since 1984 transducers were developed which can be positioned in the vagina. This brings the active transducer elements into close contact with the uterus and fetus. Higher frequencies are possible and the resolution is improved at least five fold. There are limitations in that with the higher frequency the field of view is reduced to about 8 cms. One can use a lower frequency but with a significant loss in resolution and, after all, achieving higher resolution was the original intent and advantage of this type of probe. Endovaginal or transvaginal ultrasound is now the standard for the study of the first trimester embryo and for the study of the *presenting part* of the second and third trimester fetus.

The latest development that has surfaced and brings great promise for the future is the use of very high frequency (12-15 MHz) transducers that fit inside a catheter which can be placed in almost any orifice. Studies from UCLA in Los Angeles show very promising higher resolution images of the 2 mm Stage 9 embryo using a 12 MHz catheter probe placed in the endometrial canal adjacent to the gestational sac. At this time studies are limited to women slated for therapeutic abortion. The cardiac and neural tubes are just discernable even at this early stage of six weeks menstrual age. The yolk sac is well seen and one could readily imagine that it could be punctured for the analysis of intra-sac fluid or, in turn, that fluid, chemicals or cells could be placed into the sac for incorporation into the embryo. This presents very exciting possibilities for embryos with an inborn error of metabolism. If it is detected early, it may be correctable with the installation of a group of "normal" cells into the yolk sac that would then be incorporated into the fetus creating a mosaic. This may result in a normal functioning newborn.

Being able to access the embryo in this manner opens an era of ultrahigh resolution embryonic imaging. One should be able to see exquisite anatomic detail but also to detect and record physiological events such as blood flow in the embryo and the yolk sac, and limb and body movement. But what about our present limitations in "seeing and displaying" the whole embryo or fetus? I think that there is a solution that exists within the near future–the next two to three years: three-dimensional imaging.

The Near Future

Three-dimensional (3D) imaging is here today but only in its infancy. A number of centers are now involved in credible 3D imaging research. Four equipment manufacturers have scanners that they are or will in the next six months be sending out for clinical trials. The ultimate goal is real time acquisition and display of a large field of view, all in three dimensions.

Each of these requirements poses problems with today's technology, but ones that are not insurmountable. Two-dimensional phased array transducers are being built and tested for the acquisition of the images but technically this still poses a challenge. A computer fast enough to acquire all incoming data and "large" enough to store and retrieve the data is another major challenge. Parallel processing and specially built transputers hold the promise in the near future. Finally, present day flat screen monitors are hopelessly inadquate to display an image in three dimensions. There are now 3D video display units that create what looks like a holographic image in space. This may provide an answer in the near future.

To be able to see the embryo or fetus within its natural environment in three dimensions means that we can see the gross surface morphology, the relatively large fetal head, the limbs and the body with its bulging anterior wall filled with the beating heart or the full liver. Imagine the thrill of seeing, for the first time, movement of embryonic limbs in real time 3D. Now imagine pressing a button and the embryo becomes "transparent." The beating heart and the individual chambers and valves come into view, you sweep up to the head to see the lateral ventricles filling the cranial vault in the eight-week embryo and see the echogenic choroid plexus as it, in turn, fills the ventricles. Under the influence of the vascular plexus within the choroid, it pulsates and bounces around within the cavernous ventricle. Imagine seeing the spinal cord within the vertebral column. Each of the three components of the vertebrae, the lateral masses and the body are clearly seen surrounding the cord. Surely the diagnosis of neural tube defects within the brain and spinal cord will be "child's play."

We must have the technology to allow us to see not only the small embryo but also the large, term or near-term fetus. This, in turn, presents a major challenge but, as with the other hurdles to cross, there are potential solutions. Large field transducer arrays directly applied to the abdomen may be able to encompass the second trimester fetus but unlikely the third trimester ones. One could move back in time 20 years and introduce a water bath to offset the transducer from the abdomen and allow the imaging beam to encompass the entire fetus. This would be similar to the Australian scanners of the 70's with a large metal scanning bed with a water filled chamber, at the bottom of which were eight large diameter transducers. The woman lay on her stomach on the bed while the transducers swept back and forth creating a series of two-dimensional slices or scans. If you replaced the individual transducers with two-dimensional transducer arrays and integrated ALL of the returning information, you could literally see the entire fetus and eliminate the information loss by the shadowing bones. This may be the only way to get real time 3D of large areas. It is possible, but it would be a monster and this is not what people want or will use. The Australian "dinosaur" is dead and is unlikely to reappear in the evolutionary pathway of the scanners of tomorrow.

If a transducer array had a position sensing device attached to it and were to be moved over the uterus, and if the computer could integrate all of the incoming data, then you could see the whole fetus BUT not in real time.

With real time 3D you could again watch fetal movement response to stimuli, both internal and external, and obtain a real sense of fetal well being. BUT this is part of the far future of five or more years from now.

The Far Future

Far is only a relative term. Who knows what major advances will arrive even within the next 12 months? The rapid advance of computer technology within the last five years was an exponential increase over the preceding 10 years, so "far" may be tomorrow.

What can we imagine that might make ultrasound imaging of the fetus even more exciting than some of the features we have already discussed? If we added even more physiological information, such as color-coded blood flow, you could create an even more complete "picture" of the fetus. This would, of course, all be seen in real time and in three dimensions. The only impediment is computer power and the limitation of the speed of sound. We can only transmit and receive so much ultrasound data while retaining a frame rate that approximates real time. Perhaps with more sensitive or more numerous transducer elements . . . it's hard to say. This one may be too tough, but let's challenge them to create *real time 3D images with color flow.*

Let your mind wander for a minute and consider *Virtual reality.* This is the imaging of the future and to a certain extent is here today. The recent film "Lawnmower Man" by Steven King introduced the public to the concept of "living" within a computer—being able to "see" yourself floating in computer space and to interact with the UNREAL or VIRTUAL environment or reality. In the construction industry it is being used to allow people to "walk" through a home and to "see" it as if they were actually inside. With a special headset that places small television monitors in front of your eyes and a gyroscope that senses changes in the position of your head, you can look up and "see" the ceiling, open a door, walk into a room and look around. You will see windows with light shining through depending on the "time of day" and will actually see furniture that can be moved effortlessly anywhere in space.

The fetus can be placed in virtual space and you can reach out and hold it, examine it and even look from the inside out. How best to examine the most minute details of an organ such as the heart if not as an *antemortem* pathologist who can "hold" the organ, examining it from every angle. The nicest thing is that when you are finished there is nothing to clean up or put back together.

It seems as if I let my familiarity with morphology get the best of me. I have focused on what might be needed in new equipment advances in order to see the whole fetus. On the other hand, this is really the first step to *observing* the fetus over time. In the far future I can imagine that each pregnancy will be "captured" in a movie that starts with the early embryo at six or seven weeks and follows it weekly and then monthly until delivery. The three-dimensional real time images will be joined together to provide not only an ongoing record of growth and development, but finally a complete record of a normal or abnormal outcome. Monitoring or development will involve not only a view of what the fetus is today, but how that has evolved over time. This will give us much needed insight into the processes that end in an unfavorable outcome, so that we can detect it at its earliest and deal with it in the most appropriate manner available.

As I descend from 35,000 feet, through the clouds of conjecture, it is important to remember that what we can achieve is limited only by what we can imagine. Imagine what you will and challenge those that can–I have–now let's wait and see.

Index

T - #0240 - 101024 - C0 - 212/152/13 [15] - CB - 9781560244493 - Gloss Lamination